THE DIABETES ⊦

Insulin Dependent
Diabetes

THE DIABETES HANDBOOK
Non-insulin Dependent Diabetes

Dr John L. Day M.D.,F.R.C.P.

Chairman of the BDA Education Advisory Committee

THORSONS PUBLISHING GROUP

Published in collaboration with
The British Diabetic Association
10 Queen Anne Street, London W1M 0BD

First published 1986

British Library Cataloguing in Publication Data

Day, John L.
  The diabetes handbook.
  Insulin dependent diabetes
  1. Diabetes — Treatment   2. Self-care,
  Health
  I. Title   II. British Diabetic Association
  616.4'62   RC660

  ISBN 0-7225-1370-4

Printed and bound in Singapore

10 9 8 7 6 5 4 3

Contents

Foreword

1 Introduction   1

2 Insulin dependent diabetes   11

3 Controlling your diabetes   21

4 Is your treatment effective?   63

5 Keeping perfect balance   73

6 What can go wrong?   81

7 Long-term complications   95

8 Marriage, pregnancy and contraception   107

9 Diabetes and your daily life   117

10 Diabetes in children   143

Appendix 1   How to inject insulin   169

Appendix 2   Urine tests   189

Appendix 3   Blood tests   197

Appendix 4   Treating severe hypoglycaemia with glucagon   201

Appendix 5   Food values for those with diabetes   207

Appendix 6   Insulin infusion pumps   223

Appendix 7   The child with diabetes at school —
             guidelines for teachers   225

Appendix 8   What the babysitter needs to know   227

Appendix 9   BDA publications   231

Glossary   233

Index   240

Foreword

Today people with diabetes can lead full and active lives and expect to be as healthy as people without diabetes. However, to enjoy good health with diabetes demands self-discipline, understanding and knowledge. Nobody can be expected to follow rules and recommendations without a clear explanation of the reasons for doing so.

So it is a pleasure to welcome this new British Diabetic Association Handbook. It is comprehensive and thoroughly up-to-date. It contains all the essential information.

The Handbook has been prepared by experts in the field. It is clearly and sympathetically written, copiously illustrated and well designed, so that even the most complex aspects of diabetes and its control are easy to understand. It is invaluable as a reference book and as an easy to follow practical guide to good diabetic control. Nobody with diabetes should be without it.

Sir Harry Secombe CBE

Introduction

History

The correct name for diabetes is diabetes mellitus. 'Diabetes' is derived from a Greek word meaning syphon, and 'mellitus' refers to the characteristic sweetness of the urine of those with diabetes. This title describes one of the most important features of the disease — the passage of very large amounts of sweet urine.

Diabetes is very common. In the UK there are more than 600,000 people with diabetes, of whom over 30,000 are children; world-wide there are over 30 million.

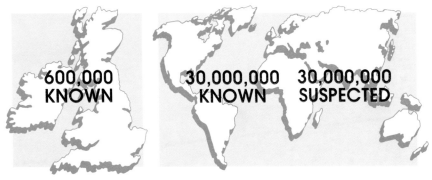

Fig. 1.1
The estimated numbers of people with diabetes.

Diabetes has been known to physicians for thousands of years, one of the first references to it being in the Ebers Papyrus (Fig. 1.2) written in Egypt in 1500BC. It is also referred to in ancient Indian, Roman, Japanese and Chinese writings. However, it was not until the last century that any significant advance was made in understanding the nature of diabetes, or in developing an effective form of treatment. The first major breakthrough came in 1889, when two German scientists discovered that the removal of the pancreas, a large gland in the abdomen, gave rise to diabetes. About this time, it was also discovered that damage to specific cells in the

Fig. 1.2
The Ebers Papyrus.

Written about 1500 BC, this is one of the earliest documents describing the treatment of diabetes. The treatment is called "A medicine to drive away the passing of too much urine . . ." and included a mixture of bones, wheat grains, fresh grits, green lead, earth and water. These ingredients the user should "let stand moist, strain it, take it for four days".

The Papyrus, measuring over 20 metres long and 30 centimetres wide, was found in a grave in Thebes in Egypt, in 1862.

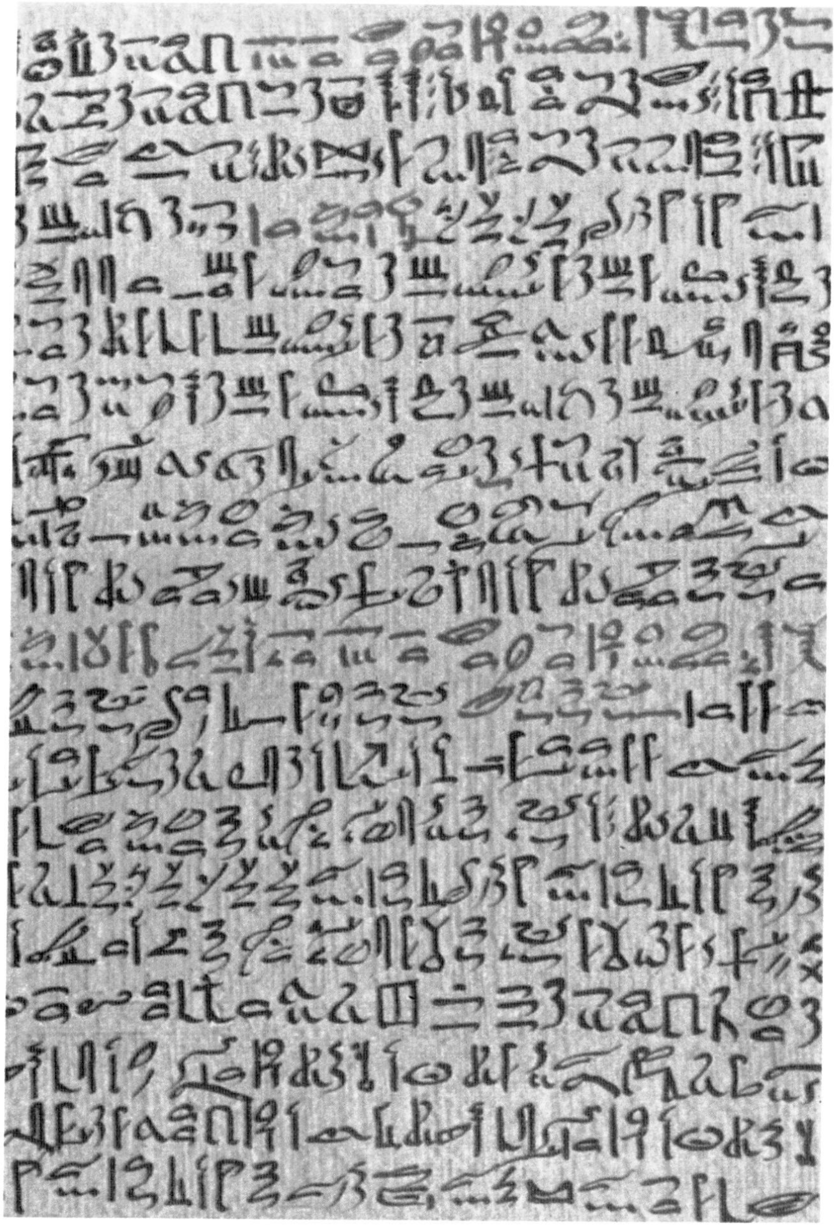

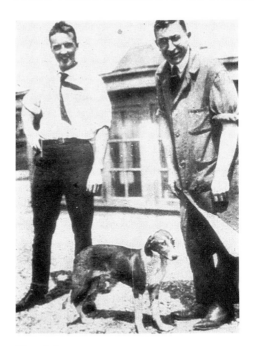

pancreas, called islets of Langerhans, produced certain forms of diabetes. But it was not until 1921 that two Canadians, Frederick Banting and Charles Best (Fig. 1.3) made their famous discovery of insulin, a hormone produced by the islets of Langerhans.

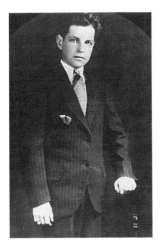

Since 1922, when they treated their first patient (Fig. 1.4), millions of lives have been saved by insulin treatment. The successful treatment of diabetes with insulin has been, without question, one of the major medical and scientific triumphs of this century.

Fig. 1.4
Leonard Thompson, the first patient with diabetes to be treated with insulin, in January 1922.

Fig. 1.3
Banting and Best.
Frederick Banting and Charles Best, whose research led to the isolation of insulin. The photograph shows them with their famous dog, Marjorie, which was kept alive by insulin after her pancreas had been removed.

Modern treatment enables many thousands of people with diabetes to achieve complete, fruitful, healthy lives and to fulfil their ambitions in all walks of life. Insulin treatment is a bar to very few jobs. People with diabetes are found amongst our most successful actors, actresses, entertainers, politicians, first-class footballers, sportsmen and sportswomen competing at the highest level, and in all the professions; all of these bear witness to the fact that effective treatment can be combined with the highest achievements.

What is diabetes?

In simple terms, diabetes is a disorder in which the body is unable to control the amount of sugar in the blood, because the mechanism which converts sugar to energy is no longer functioning properly. This leads to an abnormally high level of sugar in the blood, which gives rise to a variety of symptoms. If the sugar levels are uncontrolled over several years, it may damage various tissues of the body. Therefore, the treatment of diabetes is designed not only to reverse any symptoms you might have at the beginning, but also to prevent any serious problems developing later.

How does diabetes develop?

Normally, the amount of sugar (glucose) in the body is very carefully controlled. We obtain sugar from the food we eat, either from sweet things, or after the digestion of starch foods (carbohydrates), such as bread and potatoes. Under certain circumstances, however, sugar can be made in the body by breaking down body stores. This will occur when the food supply is reduced, or when more sugar is needed, such as following an injury or during an illness.

The conversion of sugar to energy requires the presence of the hormone insulin, which is produced by the pancreas. Insulin is released when the blood sugar rises after a meal, and its level falls when the blood sugar decreases (Fig. 1.5), for example during exercise. Therefore, it can be seen that insulin plays a vital role in maintaining the correct level of blood sugar, particularly by preventing the blood sugar from rising too high. When there is a shortage of insulin, or if the available insulin does not function correctly, then diabetes will result.

Fig. 1.5
Blood sugar and insulin levels rise and fall after each meal or snack.

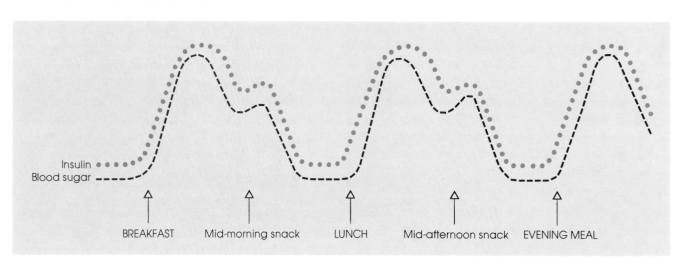

Insulin •••
Blood sugar ----

↑ BREAKFAST   ↑ Mid-morning snack   ↑ LUNCH   ↑ Mid-afternoon snack   ↑ EVENING MEAL

The consequences of diabetes are summarized below:

1. Because the blood sugar is not converted to energy, the amount of sugar in the blood builds up and spills into the urine.

2. In an attempt to compensate for the lack of energy, the liver makes much more sugar than normal.

3. Since there is an inadequate amount of insulin to convert the sugar to energy, another energy source has to be found. The body's stores of fat and protein are therefore broken down to release more sugar into the bloodstream, and there is a consequent loss of weight.

4. In the complete absence of insulin, the breakdown of fats may be excessive and substances called ketones will be found in the blood and will spill into the urine. The presence of ketones in these individuals may be demonstrated by means of urine tests. Some ketones are acids, and if very large amounts are present, as for example in severe insulin deficiency, they cause the very serious condition of diabetic keto-acidosis or diabetic coma.

Types of diabetes

There are two main types of diabetes:

1. **Insulin dependent diabetes** — also known as Type I diabetes or juvenile diabetes.

2. **Non-insulin dependent diabetes** — also known as maturity onset diabetes or Type II diabetes.

People with non-insulin dependent diabetes still produce insulin, although it may be in inadequate amounts, or it may not be working properly. They do not need to inject insulin in order to survive and, in most cases, can be treated by diet, or by a combination of diet and tablets.

Those with insulin dependent diabetes, on the other hand, because they produce little or no insulin, will not survive unless they are treated with insulin. However, not all those who take insulin are necessarily completely dependent on it, but without it perfect control of their diabetes is not possible.

The causes of diabetes and who gets it

In the United Kingdom, as many as 1 to 2 per cent of the population, and perhaps one in every 500 school children, have diabetes. It can occur at any age, but it is very rare in infants and becomes much commoner in the middle and older age groups. Amongst younger people, the sexes are almost equally affected by diabetes, whereas in older age groups, diabetes is commoner in women.

Insulin dependent diabetes

Cause

In this type of diabetes there is a complete or near complete absence of insulin, due to destruction of the insulin-producing cells of the pancreas. There is some tendency for insulin dependent diabetes to run in families, but the condition is far from being entirely inherited. The exact cause of the damage to the insulin-producing cells is not known for certain, but factors which may be involved are:

● Damage to the insulin-producing cells, as a result of viral and other infections.

● An abnormal reaction of the body against the insulin-producing cells.

Who gets it?

In general, younger people with diabetes (less than 40 years of age) are usually insulin dependent, but all age groups, even the very old, may be affected.

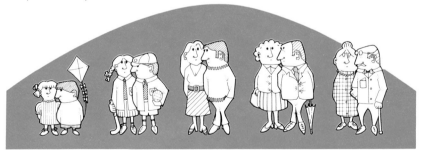

Non-insulin dependent diabetes

Cause

In this type of diabetes there is some insulin in the body, but not enough to maintain good health. The cause is not known.

Who gets it?

Non-insulin dependent diabetes used to be called 'maturity onset' diabetes, indicating that it usually occurs in the middle and older age groups, although it occasionally occurs in young people. Fat or overweight people are particularly likely to develop this type of diabetes, as are members of certain families in whom the condition is passed from one generation to the next.

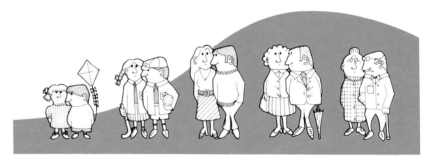

Other causes of diabetes

Diseases of the pancreas

A very few cases of diabetes are due to various diseases of the pancreas, such as inflammation of the pancreas (pancreatitis), or unusual deposits of iron. Occasionally, it occurs in rare forms of hormone imbalance.

Accidents or illnesses

Major accidents or illnesses are not thought to cause diabetes but, by causing a temporary increase in blood sugar, they may reveal pre-existing diabetes or make worse established diabetes.

If your diabetes was discovered during the course of an illness, it is highly likely that you had diabetes before the illness, even though you did not show any symptoms.

Occasionally, during very severe illnesses such as a heart attack, a serious injury, or after a major operation, the blood sugar may rise, producing a state of temporary diabetes.

Psychological stress is not believed to cause diabetes, but may certainly exacerbate it.

Drugs

Some drugs can increase the blood sugar and may reveal pre-existing diabetes. Cortisone-like (steroid) drugs commonly do this, while 'water tablets' (diuretics), which eliminate fluid from the body, do so less commonly. There are no other commonly used drugs which have this effect.

The contraceptive pill

The oral contraceptive pill does not cause diabetes, but it may raise the blood sugar slightly in those who already have the condition.

Heredity

Hereditary factors have already been briefly mentioned. The risk that the child of a father or mother who takes insulin may develop some type of diabetes before 20 years of age is higher than normal, but is still very small, probably about 1 per cent. In the rare situation where both parents have this type of diabetes, the risk is further increased, but by an uncertain amount, and professional genetic counselling may be sought.

In the more common, non-insulin dependent diabetes, the situation is somewhat different, in that the condition is predominantly inherited. Because this type of diabetes usually occurs in people who are middle-aged or older, there are relatively few women of child-bearing age with non-insulin dependent diabetes.

So, to summarize, it is possible for someone to inherit a proneness to diabetes, but not the condition itself, which will only develop as a result of the influence of some other factor. Thus, there are a large number of people who never develop diabetes, even though they have an inherited tendency to do so.

Onset of symptoms and their severity

The main symptoms of diabetes are:

- Thirst and a dry mouth
- Passing large amounts of urine
- Weight loss
- Tiredness
- Itching of the genital organs
- Blurring of vision.

Symptoms vary considerably in their severity and rate of onset, but they can all be rapidly relieved by treatment.

Insulin dependent diabetes

The condition develops fairly quickly, usually over a few weeks, but it may take as little as a few days, or as long as several months. Without insulin treatment the condition progressively worsens, resulting in a significant weight loss, dehydration, vomiting, the onset of drowsiness and diabetic coma.

Non-insulin dependent diabetes

The symptoms are similar to those of insulin dependent diabetes, but they develop more gradually and are usually less severe. Diabetic coma does not occur in this type of diabetes.

Some people with diabetes fail to notice any symptoms, but after being treated they usually have more energy and feel considerably better. Unfortunately, the presence of symptoms is no guide to the level of sugar in the blood, and it is essential that diabetes is treated, even when there are no symptoms.

Treatment

Diabetes is a very common disorder. Although no 'cure' is possible, all types of diabetes can be treated and normal health restored.

Treatment is with:

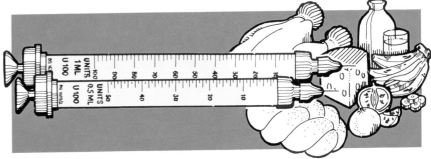

● Insulin and diet — for insulin dependent diabetes

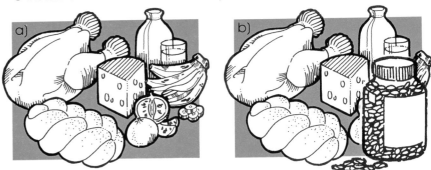

● Diet or diet and tablets — for non-insulin dependent diabetes.

Treatment must be maintained throughout life. This is necessary not only to avoid symptoms and the risk of coma, but also to minimize the risks of any later complications.

All forms of treatment require some modification to daily routines, and the performance of checks to ensure that treatment is effective. However, you should be able to achieve these with only minimal disturbance to your daily life.

From Chapter 2 onwards, this Handbook explains in detail what has gone wrong in your type of diabetes and describes how, with correct treatment, you should be able to maintain effective control.

With insulin dependent diabetes you will have been advised that you need to have regular insulin injections in order to return to, and maintain, good health. If you understand how insulin controls sugar in the body, the steps you have to take in order to control your diabetes will be much easier to follow.

Where does blood sugar come from?

Under normal circumstances the sugar in the blood comes from the food we eat:

- **Sweet things,**
  e.g. sugar added to cereals, drinks, sweets, jams, etc.
- **Starch foods,**
  e.g. bread, potatoes, cereals, flour, etc.

Fig. 2.1 shows that after a meal sugar is absorbed into the blood supply and is transported to the individual body cells, where it is used for the production of energy. Any excess sugar in the blood, which is not required for the provision of immediate energy, can be stored in either of two forms:

1. As starch (glycogen) in the liver, for later conversion back to sugar if the body needs additional energy, e.g. during exercise, at times of injury or during sickness.

   In the healthy individual, the level of blood sugar is kept within close limits, but will be at its lowest several hours after a meal, and at its highest just after a meal. The co-ordination of the overall supply of energy in the body is undertaken by the liver. In addition to its ability to provide more energy in times of special need, the liver provides from its own stores a steady trickle of sugar into the blood when you are not eating. In this way it ensures that the blood sugar level remains normal.

2. As fat (triglyceride) in the fat stores of the body.

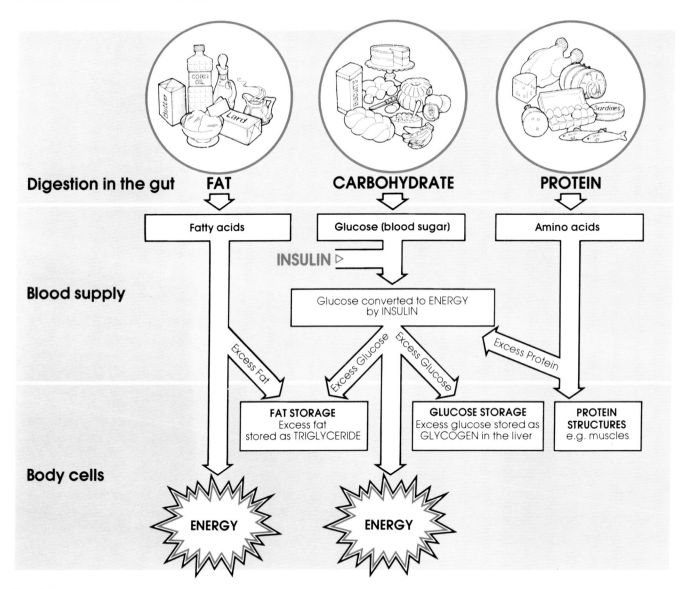

Fig. 2.1
Normal metabolism.
In the presence of insulin, glucose can be converted to energy.

Where does insulin come from?

The key to the conversion of sugar to energy, or its storage as glycogen or fat, is the hormone insulin. Insulin is produced by a gland in the abdomen, called the pancreas. As can be seen from Fig. 2.2, the pancreas contains little groups of cells, the islets of Langerhans, and it is these cells which sense the level of sugar in the blood and send just the right amount of insulin into the blood to dispose of it. In a person with diabetes, the pancreas either produces insufficient insulin to convert the glucose to energy, fat or glycogen (as happens with non-insulin dependent diabetes), or if the islets have been damaged, it produces little or none at all. This is the situation which exists in insulin dependent diabetes and is the reason why it is necessary to inject insulin regularly, in order to control the blood sugar level.

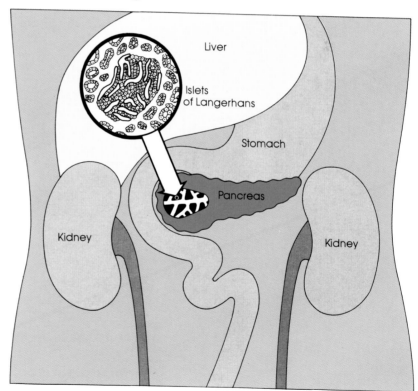

Fig. 2.2
The pancreas.
The pancreas is a large gland positioned behind the stomach. The inset shows the detailed structure of the insulin-producing cells, the islets of Langerhans.

How does insulin work?

Whenever we eat, the blood sugar rises. This is the signal for insulin to go into action. Normally, insulin pours out of the pancreas during the half hour after a meal.

Fig. 2.3 shows the blood sugar rising after a meal. As soon as the glucose begins to rise, the pancreas detects the change and immediately starts releasing insulin into the blood, as shown in Fig. 2.4. As the insulin speeds through the circulation, it allows sugar to penetrate into the body cells, so that about two hours after a meal, the blood sugar falls back to the fasting level.

Fig. 2.3
Blood sugar rising during the half hour after a meal.

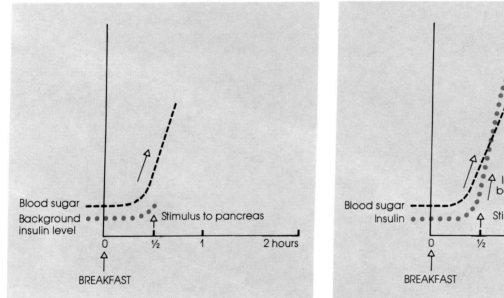

Fig. 2.4
Insulin released from the pancreas makes the blood sugar level fall.

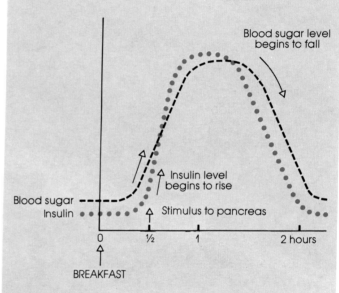

Thus, there are two important facts to remember:

1 The blood sugar rises after each meal.

2 Insulin brings the sugar level down to normal.

Fig. 2.5
Insulin levels keep closely in step with
sugar levels throughout the day.

Whenever we eat, the blood sugar rises and it is at this time,
therefore, that we need an extra boost of insulin to convert the
sugar to energy, and thus make it available for use by the body

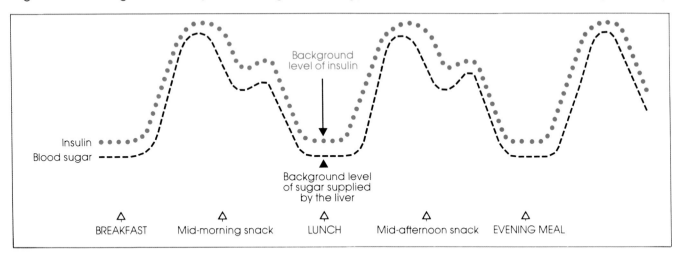

Background
level of insulin

Insulin
Blood sugar

Background level
of sugar supplied
by the liver

BREAKFAST   Mid-morning snack   LUNCH   Mid-afternoon snack   EVENING MEAL

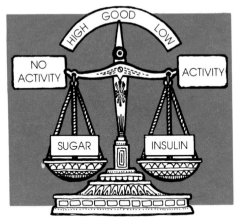

Fig. 2.6
Control = Balance.

Good control of blood sugar depends on a
balance between the sugar from the diet and
the amount of insulin produced. This balance
can be altered by the effects of exercise, or
lack of it.

cells. Insulin production keeps very closely in step with sugar levels,
as can be seen from Fig. 2.5. It is important to appreciate that these
are extra boosts of insulin, and that between meals there is always
a steady background release of insulin. This insulin converts the
steady trickle of sugar supplied by the liver into energy, thus
enabling the cells to keep 'ticking over'.

Effect of exercise

During heavy work or exercise, more energy is required. This calls
for an increased supply of sugar, and its conversion to energy.
Normally, the blood sugar is prevented from falling too low by
receiving a top-up from the liver. If, however, the insulin level should
be too high, as can occur in those who inject insulin, the liver
may not be able to keep up its supply of sugar and consequently
the blood sugar falls. We call this state of low blood sugar
'hypoglycaemia' (hypo = low, glyc = sugar, aemia = in the blood).
Exercise can cause hypoglycaemia. Thus, control of the blood
sugar depends on a 'balance' between the supply of sugar from

food or the liver and its disposal as energy or stored energy. This balance, which depends directly on the amount of insulin available, is summarized in Fig. 2.6.

What happens without insulin?

The blood sugar rises

Without insulin the body is unable to burn up the energy it needs or to store it, with the result that the blood sugar increases. This increase occurs between meals, but climbs even higher just after meals. The situation is made worse by the fact that the liver is no longer under proper control and, as a result, releases its stored sugar. The net result is an even greater build up of blood sugar (hyperglycaemia).

Sugar in the urine

Normally, the filtering effect of the kidneys prevents the passage of sugar into the urine. When there is too little insulin, however, the blood sugar can reach a certain level — the 'renal threshold' (Fig. 2.7) — at which point it starts to spill over into the urine (Fig. 2.8) in ever-increasing quantities (glycosuria). This gives rise to three of the commonest symptoms of uncontrolled diabetes:

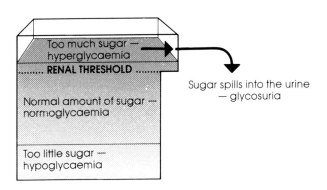

Fig. 2.7
Blood sugar levels.

When the blood sugar reaches a certain level it spills over into the urine. This level is called the renal threshold.

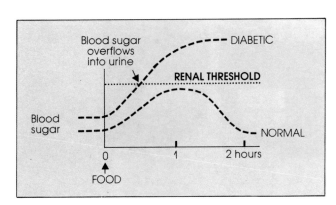

Fig. 2.8
Glycosuria.

The blood sugar rises above the renal threshold because of a lack of insulin, and spills over into the urine.

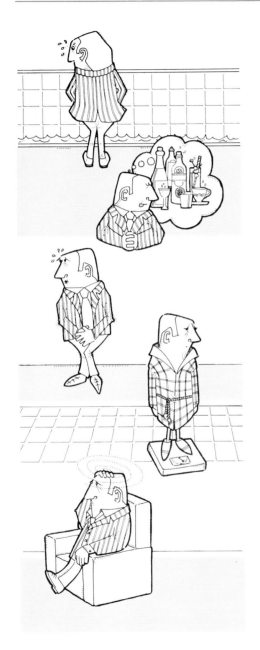

● Passing large quantities of urine

In order to get rid of the excess sugar, more water is excreted by the kidneys, and this results in the frequent passing of large volumes of urine. This can give rise to bed-wetting in some children, and incontinence in the elderly.

● Thirst

Because more water is leaving the body, a dry mouth and a feeling of thirstiness may develop. It will actually be made worse by drinking soft drinks, which contain a lot of sugar.

● Genital soreness

When large quantities of sugar are passed in the urine, it tends to create soreness around the genital area. It frequently causes itching of the vulva in women (in whom thrush is more likely to develop) and, less frequently, it produces itching of the penis in men. Once diabetes is controlled and sugar disappears from the urine, these unpleasant problems rapidly disappear.

Breakdown of body energy stores

Because a shortage or absence of insulin prevents blood sugar from being converted into energy, an energy source must be provided from elsewhere (Fig. 2.9). Consequently, there is a breakdown of fat and protein (muscle), which results in:

● Weight loss

Diabetes is one of the commonest causes of weight loss, and occurs in most people at the onset of the disorder. It ranges from a few pounds to two or three stone in some of the more severe cases.

● Tiredness and weakness

Tiredness, often accompanied by a sensation of weakness, is very common in uncontrolled diabetes. Some people are more than usually prone to fall asleep at odd times, while others just feel they are growing old before their time. This symptom can, of course, be completely reversed by treatment. Many feel

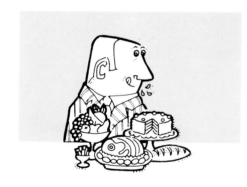

'rejuvenated' after starting a course of treatment, even when they had previously been unaware of any abnormalities.

- **An increased appetite**

In some individuals there is a noticeable increase in appetite.

Keto-acidosis

Keto-acidosis (also called ketosis or diabetic coma) is a complication of insulin deficiency which <u>must be avoided</u> at all costs. It is caused by a lack of insulin, or when the body's need for insulin is increased, such as during an infection or an illness.

In the absence of insulin the liver, besides swamping the blood with sugar, tries to replace this fuel by breaking down fat (Fig. 2.9). As a result, breakdown products called ketones are made, and although not harmful in small quantities, in large amounts they are poisonous acids. One of the ketones, called acetone, which smells like nail varnish remover, can be detected on the breath of some people with uncontrolled diabetes.

Ketones are danger signals, indicating virtual absence of insulin. With the right amount of insulin, the blood sugar can be lowered, and ketones eliminated. When there is a severe lack of insulin, large amounts of ketones give rise to the very serious condition of diabetic keto-acidosis or diabetic coma. This is particularly likely to occur if insulin is reduced or stopped, or if you are vomiting or ill; it does not occur if you are eating and drinking normally.

Symptoms of this condition include:

- Confusion
- Nausea
- Weakness
- Vomiting
- Increased passage of urine
- Abdominal upsets
- Thirstiness
- Shortness of breath

If ketosis remains untreated — and hospital treatment is always essential when this state has been reached — diabetic coma will follow. Prior to the availability of insulin, this was always fatal.

Fig. 2.9
Breakdown of body energy stores.
Because of a shortage of insulin and a consequent shortage of energy, alternative energy sources are provided by the breakdown of body energy stores (compare with Fig. 2.1).

Remember, once you have started insulin treatment, it should NEVER be stopped. Therefore, it is absolutely ESSENTIAL that you PREVENT the risk of ketosis by taking enough insulin. Also, because illness can cause ketosis, you should read carefully the section on how to deal with your diabetes when you are unwell, Chapter 6, page 82.

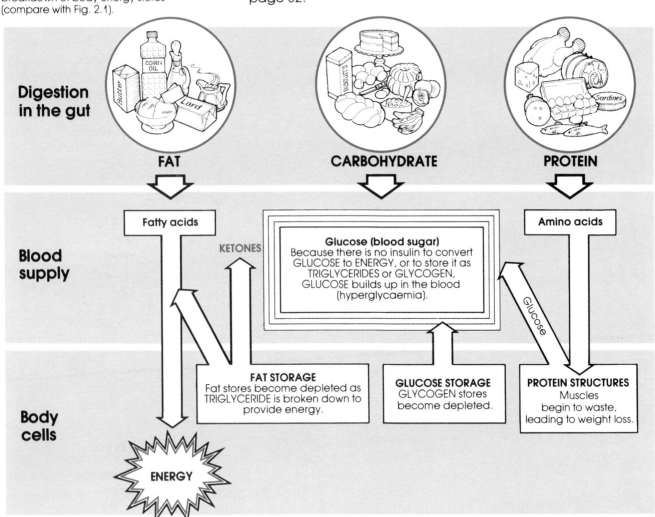

Digestion in the gut

FAT   CARBOHYDRATE   PROTEIN

Blood supply

Fatty acids

KETONES

Amino acids

Glucose

Glucose (blood sugar)
Because there is no insulin to convert GLUCOSE to ENERGY, or to store it as TRIGLYCERIDES or GLYCOGEN, GLUCOSE builds up in the blood (hyperglycaemia).

Body cells

FAT STORAGE
Fat stores become depleted as TRIGLYCERIDE is broken down to provide energy.

GLUCOSE STORAGE
GLYCOGEN stores become depleted.

PROTEIN STRUCTURES
Muscles begin to waste, leading to weight loss.

ENERGY

Other effects of high blood sugar

These include:

● **Infections**

In the presence of high blood sugar, some other mechanisms in the body may not function as well as they should. During such periods you may be more prone to infections, such as abscesses, whitlows or urinary infections.

● **Blurring of vision**

The high level of sugar in the body causes the lens of the eye to change slightly in shape. Consequently, short-sightedness is sometimes experienced when diabetes develops, but the reverse sometimes occurs, making reading difficult. These changes may only be noticed in the early stages of treatment, and normally sight is completely restored in two or three weeks. It is wise, however, not to have your eyes tested for new glasses for at least one month after proper stabilization of the diabetes.

Long-term effects of diabetes

Over a long period of time, a high blood sugar — even if it is not causing symptoms — will damage the small blood vessels in a number of tissues, the most commonly affected being:

● The eyes — perhaps causing loss of vision
● The nerves — causing numbness or painful tingling
● The kidneys
● The feet — especially in the elderly.

These are the so-called 'long-term' or 'late' complications of diabetes, and are discussed in more detail in Chapter 7, page 95.

It must be stressed that these complications will develop <u>only</u> if a high blood sugar is sustained over a period of several years. Therefore, if your blood sugar can be returned to normal and you can maintain good control, then the risks of complications developing are minimized.

The only way to eliminate symptoms, prevent ketosis, and minimize late complications, is to commence treatment as soon as possible and to maintain it without interruption, keeping your blood sugar as close to normal as possible.

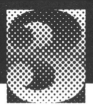

Controlling your diabetes

Aims of treatment

The two mains aims of treatment are to:
1. Eliminate symptoms.
2. Prevent late complications.

Eliminating symptoms

The first aim of treatment is to eliminate your symptoms, by returning your blood sugar level to normal. Once treatment has started, your feeling of well-being will be restored, and, as long as treatment is continued, there should be no recurrence of symptoms.

Preventing late complications

If your blood sugar is returned to normal and kept there most of the time, the risk of complications will be very slight. Your treatment must be individually tailored to suit you. The success of your treatment will depend on your ability to persevere with the prescribed treatment. Initially, this may take some getting used to. However, if you can understand the reasons for your treatment, and recognize the factors which contribute to fluctuations in your day-to-day blood sugar levels, such as your eating, working and exercise patterns, you can adjust your treatment accordingly, and maintain good control. In this way, what at first seems like a major upset to your life will quickly become a normal and unobtrusive part of your daily routine.

Unfortunately, there is no cure for diabetes, so the treatment pattern you establish must be continued for life.

In summary, the general principles of your treatment are four-fold:
1. You must take insulin injections to replace the insulin which you are failing to produce naturally — your insulin must never be stopped.
2. You must restore the balance between 'sugar-in' and 'sugar-out'. This will require you to make adjustments to the type and

amount of food you eat, and when you eat it.

3. You must take some exercise if you are physically able to do so.

4. You must make certain checks that your treatment is effective.

The first three principles of treatment will be considered in more detail in this chapter, while checking that your treatment is effective will form the subject of Chapter 4, page 63.

INSULIN
Injections of insulin

Unfortunately, there is no other way of giving insulin except by injection. Insulin cannot be given by mouth because it is a protein-like substance, which is destroyed in the stomach.

Initially, most people are apprehensive about having to inject themselves or their children with insulin once or twice a day. However, the majority of people find the procedure to be simpler and much less painful than they first imagined.

Full details of all you need to know about injections are given in Appendix 1, page 169.

Insulin and restoring the balance

During the first few days of insulin injections, the aim will be to establish a balance between the insulin and blood sugar. As each individual differs, blood sugar tests will have to be performed — perhaps several times a day — to make sure that you have neither too much nor too little insulin. The point to remember is that you are trying to achieve small rises and falls in the sugar level in your blood, similar to those occurring normally. Your aim is to avoid wide swings in the blood sugar level, and so restore and maintain a state of balance.

Several factors may influence this balance:

- The type of insulin you inject
- The time of day you inject your insulin
- The times at which you eat your meals
- The amount and type of food you eat
- The frequency, timing and quantity of exercise you take.

Types of insulin

Fig. 3.1.
Insulin is produced after each meal or snack.

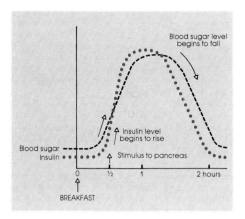

There are many types of insulin, each with different characteristics and varying durations of action. Insulin is obtained from the pancreas of animals (beef or pig); more recently, human insulin has been made in the laboratory (this is not extracted from human pancreas). The various insulins have minor differences in chemical structure, but they all work the same way.

When the pancreas is working normally, it produces short spurts or peaks of insulin in the blood, after each meal or snack (Fig. 3.1). However, when insulin is injected, its effectiveness may last for only a few hours, which means that an injection given after breakfast may no longer be active after lunch. Since the discovery of insulin, attempts have been made to change its characteristics, with the result that some insulins are effective shortly after being injected, while others have a delayed action. Thus, by choosing the right type of insulin or mixture of insulins for you, normal, balanced spurts or peaks of insulin can be achieved, and control of your diabetes can be maintained.

So, which insulin is best for you? This is a difficult question to answer, because some insulins work better and last for longer or shorter periods in different people. It is very much a matter of which insulin best suits <u>you</u> — there are no firm rules which indicate that you <u>must</u> have one type of insulin as opposed to another. In all cases, the choice is made by your doctor.

Clear and cloudy insulins

The various types of insulin can be divided into two kinds according to their appearance:

1. CLEAR

2. CLOUDY (sometimes called 'turbid')

To enable you to check which insulins are which, a list is given in Table 1.

TABLE 1 Insulins

CLEAR	CLOUDY		
Neutral insulin injection	Isophane insulin injection	Neuphane	Tempulin
Actrapid MC	Human Monotard	Rapitard MC*	Semitard
Human Actrapid	Human Ultratard	Human Initard 50/50*	Ultratard MC
Human Velosulin	Human Protaphane	Hypurin lente	Human Mixtard 30/70*
Humulin S	Humulin I	Lentard MC	Initard 50/50*
Hypurin Neutral	Hypurin Isophane	Hypurin Protamine zinc	Mixtard 30/70*
Neusulin	Insulatard	Monotard MC	
Quicksol	Monophane	Neulente	
Velosulin			

*In these types of insulin, CLEAR (quick) and CLOUDY (slow) are mixed in the vial before use. These will look cloudy.

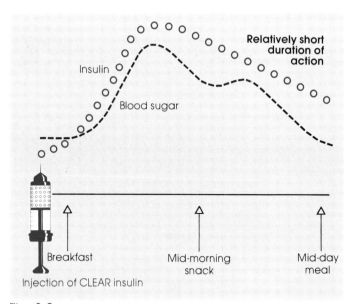

Fig. 3.2.
Clear insulin.
Clear insulin is quick-acting and has a relatively short duration of action.

Clear insulin

CLEAR insulin is quick-acting, having a relatively short duration of action of 8 to 10 hours. When injected before breakfast, it is absorbed fairly quickly, so that it builds up in the blood, reaching its peak an hour or two after breakfast (Fig. 3.2).

You will remember, that when the pancreas is working normally and producing its own insulin, the insulin level is highest when the sugar is highest, i.e. after a meal (see Fig. 2.5). Thus, with quick-acting insulin, most of the dose is available when it is most needed, namely, when the sugar has built up after breakfast.

But, does this mean that an injection is necessary before every meal? Fortunately not. This is where CLOUDY insulin comes in.

Cloudy insulin

CLOUDY insulin is slow-acting, the effects usually lasting for 12 to 14 hours, although some types last for 24 hours. If it is injected before breakfast, very little gets into the blood until lunchtime, when it builds up to a peak to coincide with the rise in blood sugar which follows the mid-day meal (Fig. 3.3). Of course, some insulin does enter the blood stream earlier than this and remains there until late afternoon, thereby providing a small amount of insulin between the peak levels which occur after meals. Remember, the pancreas supplies peak levels of insulin immediately after meals and a background level between meals. CLOUDY insulin is good for providing the trickle or background level, in order to hold the blood sugar steady between meals.

Fig. 3.3
Cloudy insulin.
Cloudy insulin is slow-acting and has a relatively long duration of action.

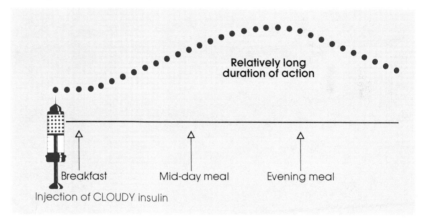

The dose of insulin

Although CLEAR is quick and CLOUDY is slow, there is another factor affecting their actions — dose.

The points to remember are that:

● If the blood sugar is consistently high, larger doses of insulin are required.

● If the blood sugar is too low, smaller doses are required.

● The bigger the dose, the higher the level of insulin in the blood and the longer it takes to disappear, i.e. it lasts longer:

i. A <u>large</u> dose of CLEAR insulin lasts longer than a <u>small</u> dose.

ii. A <u>large</u> dose of CLEAR insulin lasts nearly as long as a <u>small</u> dose of CLOUDY insulin.

This may seem very confusing, but once you know how to juggle with these facts — your doctor will give you all the advice you need — you will find that you are able to cope with almost any situation.

How insulins are used

CLEAR and CLOUDY insulins can be used in many different ways to control diabetes. Although the pancreas may not be producing any insulin when injections are started, it may recover sufficiently to produce some insulin of its own. Thus, the background levels of insulin which are provided by CLOUDY insulin, may be boosted by pancreatic insulin at mealtimes. Consequently some may manage quite well on one daily injection of CLOUDY insulin which, although it provides a reasonable amount of background insulin, does not produce much of a peak (Fig. 3.3). For others, an injection of CLEAR insulin before breakfast will provide adequate levels in the blood to cope with peaks of sugar after breakfast and after lunch, with a second injection before tea or supper to last through the night (Fig. 3.4).

Fig. 3.4
Twice-daily injections of a clear insulin.

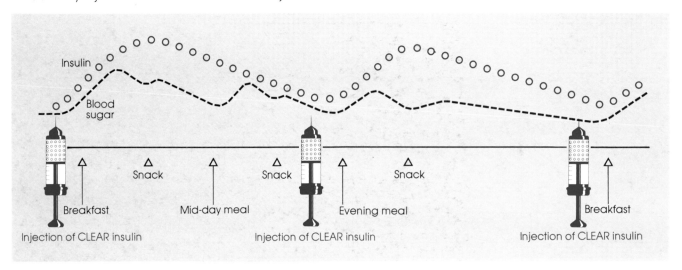

Insulin

Blood sugar

Snack   Snack   Snack

Breakfast   Mid-day meal   Evening meal   Breakfast

Injection of CLEAR insulin   Injection of CLEAR insulin   Injection of CLEAR insulin

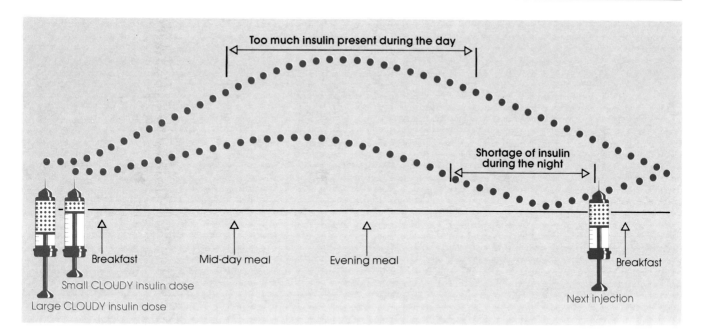

Fig. 3.5
What happens if the single, daily dose of cloudy insulin is too large or too small and little or no insulin is being produced?

In the case of those producing little or no insulin, then an inadequate dose of CLOUDY insulin in the morning will result in a shortage of insulin during the night (Fig. 3.5). However, if the insulin dose is increased in the morning, in order to produce higher levels during the evening and night, there may be too much present during the day (Fig. 3.5). This problem may be easily overcome by simply dividing this single dose of CLOUDY insulin into two equal-sized injections. As Fig. 3.6 shows, <u>smaller</u> doses are <u>shorter-acting.</u>

Many people might prefer to only give one injection but most need two or more injections, in order to get the necessary peaks of action.

One very effective way of getting these peaks and keeping a steady background trickle, is to take two injections, each combining CLEAR and CLOUDY insulin. This adds up to four insulins, each providing approximately a quarter of the daily requirement — <u>small</u> doses are <u>shorter-acting.</u> The effect of this type of dosage can be seen in Fig. 3.7. An injection taken before breakfast,

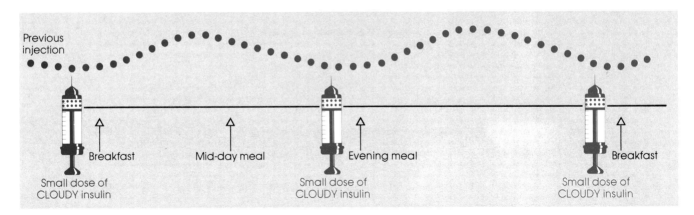

Previous injection

Breakfast   Mid-day meal   Evening meal   Breakfast

Small dose of CLOUDY insulin   Small dose of CLOUDY insulin   Small dose of CLOUDY insulin

Fig. 3.6
Smaller doses of cloudy insulin are shorter-acting than a single, daily dose.
By giving two injections it is possible to ensure the necessary levels of insulin later in the day.

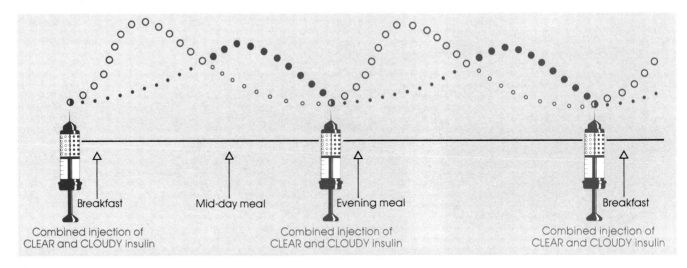

Breakfast   Mid-day meal   Evening meal   Breakfast

Combined injection of CLEAR and CLOUDY insulin   Combined injection of CLEAR and CLOUDY insulin   Combined injection of CLEAR and CLOUDY insulin

Fig.3.7
A combination of clear and cloudy insulins ensures peak as well as background levels of insulin.

combining CLEAR and CLOUDY insulins, will provide an initial peak of CLEAR insulin after breakfast and peak of CLOUDY insulin after lunch. By repeating this combination before the evening meal, the CLEAR insulin will give a peak after the meal, while the CLOUDY insulin will cover a bedtime snack and provide overnight background action.

Although once daily CLOUDY and twice daily CLEAR + CLOUDY have been described, there are several other variations which can be employed to suit an individual's way of life and eating pattern, e.g.:

- CLOUDY insulin once daily

- CLEAR insulin twice daily

- CLOUDY insulin twice daily

- CLEAR + CLOUDY insulin twice daily

- CLOUDY insulin once daily, CLEAR insulin twice daily

- Several injections of CLEAR insulin daily.

Timing of insulin injections

The aim of treatment is to keep the BLOOD INSULIN level in step with the rises in BLOOD SUGAR level after each meal, and to provide a trickle of BACKGROUND INSULIN between meals.

Most people need two injections a day. The first needs to be given at least half an hour before breakfast, and the second half an hour before the evening meal. If you have only one injection a day, then this should be given at least half an hour before breakfast. This half hour delay between injection and eating is required in order to allow the insulin to get from the injection site into the blood stream.

More details of changes in the size of the insulin dose, and in the timing of the dose, are given in Chapter 5, page 73.

Fig. 3.8
The timing of meals in relation to
insulin injections.

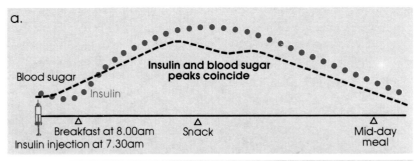

a. Meal taken at least half an hour after insulin injection.

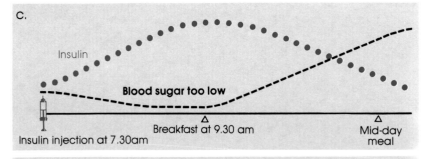

b. Meal taken only a few minutes after insulin injection.

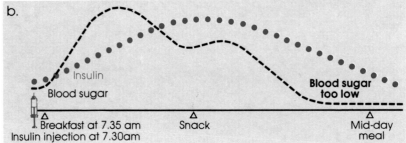

c. Meal delayed for 2 hours after insulin injection.

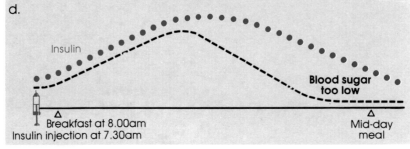

d. Mid-morning snack omitted.

Timing of meals

Meals provide the blood sugar peaks already referred to. Therefore, the timing of meals in relation to your insulin injections is of vital importance. Blood sugar control will only be achieved if the peak levels of insulin in the blood <u>coincide</u> with the peak levels of sugar (Fig. 3.8a). If you inject your insulin only a few minutes before your meal, the insulin peak will occur some time after your sugar peak, due to the time taken for the insulin to be absorbed. This may result in a high mid-morning sugar and a low late morning sugar (Fig. 3.8b). If after having injected your insulin you delay eating your meal by, say, two hours, the insulin peak will occur well before the sugar peak (Fig. 3.8c).

To ensure good control, it is essential that you should also take regular snacks. The reason for this is that if the insulin stays high when there is little or no sugar entering the circulation, i.e. before and in between meals, the insulin will cause the background sugar level to fall too low, (Fig. 3.8d). If, however, a snack is taken between meals, then the insulin and blood sugar peaks keep more closely in step. Too low a blood sugar (hypoglycaemia) is then avoided.

Infusion pumps

A recent development is the battery driven infusion pump (Fig. 3.9). The pump is worn on a belt or holster, and delivers the insulin via a fine tube connected to a needle left under the skin of the abdomen. The infusion pump has the advantage that it delivers both peak and background levels of insulin with each meal. Unfortunately, the use of infusion pumps poses special problems, and at present they are suitable only for those having particular difficulties with their diabetes. Consequently, they are not usually recommended for those whose diabetes is well controlled using traditional methods.

If you have been prescribed a pump, then you will find more details in Appendix 6, page 223.

Fig. 3.9
Insulin infusion pump.

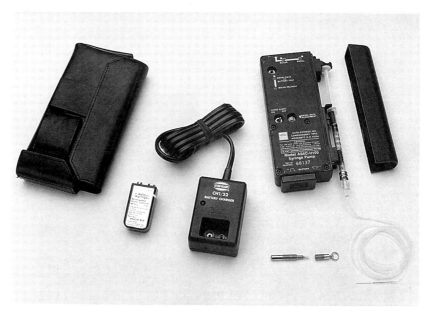

a. Components of a complete kit

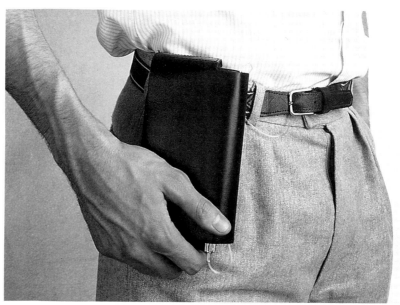

b. Infusion pump being worn on a belt.

DIET

Although you maintain control of your diabetes by injecting insulin, the type and quantity of food you eat is also of great importance if your injections are going to be effective. The relationship between blood sugar peaks and insulin peaks has already been stressed. Because the sugar peaks depend on the amount and type of food you eat and the times at which you eat, achieving the correct 'balance' in your diet is essential. To do this effectively you must have a basic knowledge of food and how it is broken down and used by the body.

The basic components of food

Our food is made up of three basic components, namely carbohydrates, fats and proteins (Fig. 3.10). All of these are essential for a balanced diet, and for the provision of energy. Many foods contain mixtures of one or more constituents. For example, milk is made up of carbohydrate, protein and fat; eggs contain fat and protein; and pastry is mainly fat and carbohydrate. In some foods, certain constituents are present only in small quantities, or are totally absent, e.g. vegetables and fruit contain little or no fat, and some dairy products, such as cheese, contain no carbohydrate.

Fig. 3.10
The three basic constituents of food.

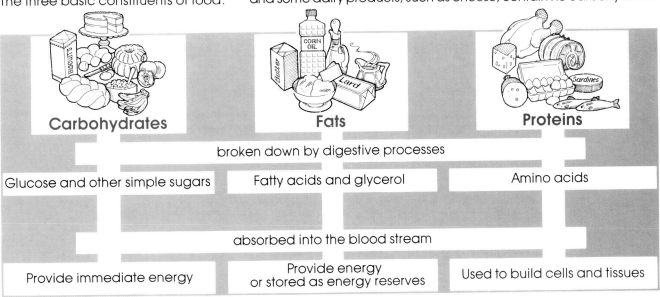

Carbohydrates	Fats	Proteins
broken down by digestive processes		
Glucose and other simple sugars	Fatty acids and glycerol	Amino acids
absorbed into the blood stream		
Provide immediate energy	Provide energy or stored as energy reserves	Used to build cells and tissues

Carbohydrate

Carbohydrate is the immediate source of sugar in the diet. The more carbohydrate you eat with a meal, the higher the level of blood sugar will be after the meal. With diabetes, this means that if you eat too much carbohydrate, you need more insulin in order to achieve the higher insulin peaks required to cope with the extra-high blood sugar level.

Carbohydrate is found in two types of food:

1. **Starchy foods**

   These have to be digested before they give rise to sugar in the blood. This process takes place fairly slowly and produces moderate and easily controllable increases in the blood sugar, when the foods contain large amounts of fibre.

   Some typical starch-containing foods include: potatoes, cereals, flour, pastries, some vegetables and fruit (Fig. 3.11). Sugar is also present in milk (lactose) and fruit (fructose)

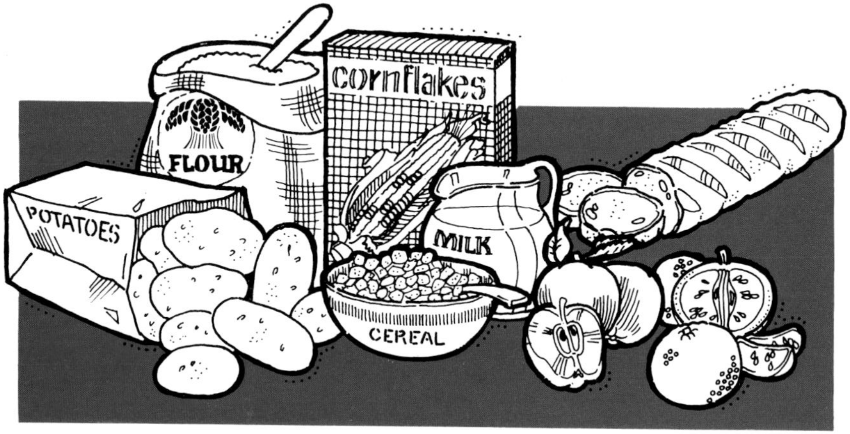

Fig. 3.11
Carbohydrates: some typical starch-containing foods.

2. **Foods containing large amounts of sugar**

   Foods containing a large amount of sugar do not require much digestion and they are therefore passed quickly into the blood-stream, giving rise to a very rapid and large increase in blood sugar. This increase may be short-lived and can produce wide

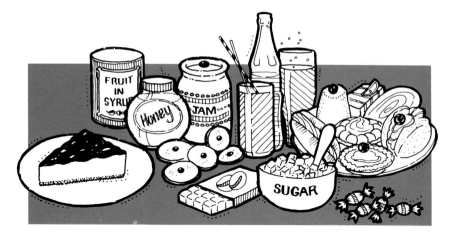

Fig. 3.12
Carbohydrates: some typical foods containing large amounts of sugar.

swings from high to low. The situation is very difficult to control with injected insulin, and achieving a balance between blood sugar and insulin levels is almost impossible.

Sugar-containing foods include honey, instant desserts, jams, soft drinks, and sweets (Fig. 3.12). Wherever possible, they are best avoided and should only be used in emergencies, when a quick rise in blood sugar is needed (see hypoglycaemia, Chapter 6, page 85).

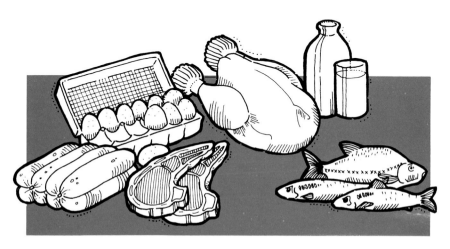

Fig. 3.13
Common foods containing protein.

Fig. 3.14
Common foods containing a lot
of fat.

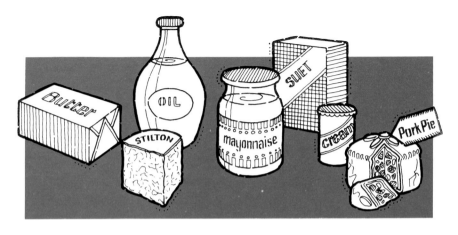

Protein

Protein is provided by meat, eggs, fish, dairy products and some vegetables (Fig. 3.13). Some protein is essential, because it provides the building materials for the cells and tissues of the body.

Fat

Some fat (Fig. 3.14) is required in the diet, but surprisingly little is necessary; even a small quantity contains a large number of calories.

Other important components of the diet

Minerals and vitamins

With the right balance of fat, carbohydrate and protein, the essential minerals and vitamins will be automatically included in the diet and supplements should not be necessary.

Fibre

This provides much of the bulk of most vegetables, some fruit, and unrefined cereal. Unfortunately, much of the fibre may be removed during modern food processing, a good example being the making of white flour. Fibre is particularly valuable as it slows down the absorption of sugar.

Planning your diet

The main aim of planning your diet is to ensure that it is BALANCED — i.e. a mixture of carbohydrate, fat and protein should be eaten which not only satisfies you, but also maintains the careful control of your diabetes. You will also learn to select foods capable of satisfying sudden energy requirements, such as occur with very strenuous work or sporting activities.

Six major factors have to be taken into account when planning your diet:

1. When and how often will you need to eat?

2. What is your total food requirement?

3. Which are the best foods to ensure good control of your diabetes?

4. Which foods should be avoided?

5. Which foods can be eaten in any amount without harm?

6. What are your tastes?

Adjusting your intake of carbohydrate

The most significant adjustments you will need to make to your diet relate to the type, amount and timing of your intake of carbohydrate.

Timing of meals

Some carbohydrate will be required for:

BREAKFAST
Mid-morning snack
MID-DAY MEAL
Afternoon snack
EVENING MEAL
Pre-bedtime snack.

The need for snacks between meals is important. At such times, you will still have insulin in your bloodstream, and therefore you will usually need to top-up the sugar level with a snack, in order to prevent it from falling too low.

The times at which you eat your meals and snacks will depend on your normal daily routine. Variations in your eating pattern will, of course be necessary, for example if you work shifts, or if you should choose to eat a meal later or earlier than usual. This is perfectly acceptable, but **YOU MUST NOT MISS OUT MEALS.** And, remember, if you vary the time of a meal, then you <u>must</u> vary the time of your insulin injection, so that the peak insulin level is reached at the <u>same</u> time as the peak sugar level.

How much carbohydrate?

The first point to remember, is that your diet must contain enough sugar to ensure a reasonable level of blood sugar, in order to provide the fuel your body needs. You **MUST NOT CUT OUT ALL FOODS PROVIDING SUGAR,** in the hope that you might not need insulin. This would merely induce your body to make more sugar from its reserves, thereby causing you to lose weight and become unwell. Starvation is no treatment for any type of diabetes.

The total amount of carbohydrate you need will be determined for you. This will be subdivided, so that you take most of it at main meals and smaller amounts at snack times.

To help you control your carbohydrate intake and still enjoy a varied and interesting diet, a system of exchanges (also called 'portions', 'rations' or 'lines') is used. If you look at Table 2, page 40, carbohydrates have been listed in single household measures, i.e. tablespoons, cups, slices etc., so that each measure of whichever type of food you prefer contains 10g of carbohydrate, called a 'portion' or an 'exchange'. All of these are equivalent (Fig. 3.15). Thus, one Weetabix is equivalent to one thin slice of bread, one egg-sized potato or two tablespoons of flour. A more detailed list is given in Appendix 5, page 207. If it has been decided that you need 5 portions for each main meal, you can then simply select those you prefer, e.g. 2 portions of bread, 2 of cereal and 1 of fruit, or any other mixture. Your snacks can be similarly varied. In these calculations you should not forget additions, such as milk with cereal.

Fig. 3.15
Some examples of foods containing
10g (1 'exchange') of carbohydrate.

It is not necessary to weigh food. With the help of lists and advice from your dietitian, you should not find difficulty in basing your quantities on household measures.

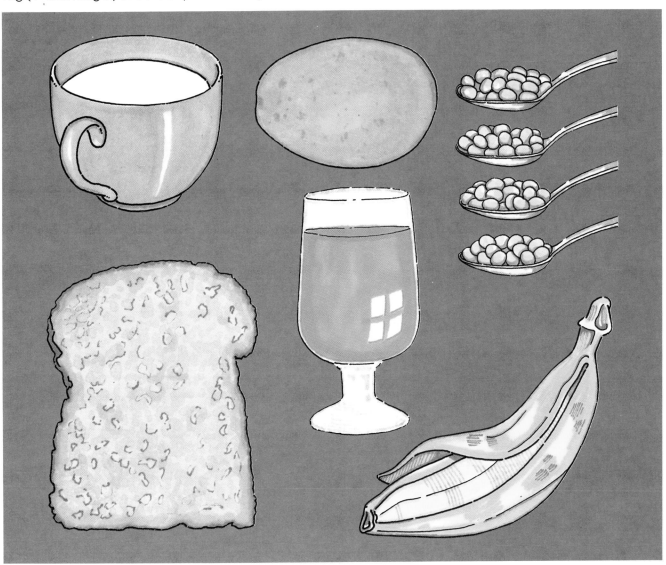

TABLE 2 Carbohydrate exchanges [†]

Foods in this list contain carbohydrate (starch) in substantial amounts.

These foods are listed in exchanges, which are equal in carbohydrate value, so you may "exchange" any of these for another on your daily menu.

Each exchange = 10g of carbohydrate

High-fibre foods are marked : * good fibre content
** very good fibre content

Spoon measures are standard kitchen spoons.

Bread and biscuits
* 1 small slice of wholemeal bread [††]
* ½ large thick slice of bread [††]
* 1 small roll [††]
2 crispbreads
* 1 digestive or wholemeal biscuit
2 cream crackers or water biscuits
2 plain or semi-sweet biscuits

Cereals
** 2 level tablespoons wholemeal flour
1½ level tablespoons white flour
** 3 level tablespoons uncooked porridge
4 tablespoons wholemeal breakfast cereal, e.g. ** Branflakes
** Shreddies
** 1 Weetabix or ⅔ Shredded Wheat
2 tablespoons cooked pasta, e.g. macaroni
2 level tablespoons cooked rice
1 level tablespoon custard powder
2 level teaspoons sago/tapioca/semolina

Choose wholemeal bread, wholewheat pasta or brown rice where possible, as they are rich in fibre.

Vegetables

** 4 level tablespoons baked beans
** 2 level tablespoons lentils (before cooking)
** 4 level tablespoons tinned or well cooked "dried" beans
2 small beetroots
1 small parsnip
1 egg-sized potato (boiled or roast)
1 scoop mashed potato
* 1 small jacket potato
* ½ medium corn-on-the-cob
* 5 tablespoons sweetcorn

Fruit

1 apple, 1 orange, 1 pear, 1 peach, 1 small banana, 10 grapes, 12 cherries, 2 dessert plums, ** 2 large prunes, 1 slice of pineapple, 15 strawberries, 2 tangerines
* 2 level tablespoons currants, raisins or sultanas
1 small bowl stewed fruit
1 small glass (4 fluid oz) fruit juice, (e.g. apple, grapefruit, orange, pineapple)
4-6 chestnuts

Milk

1 cup (⅓ pint) whole or skimmed milk
1 carton (small) plain yoghurt or ½ carton fruit yoghurt
6 tablespoons (3 fluid oz) evaporated milk

Miscellaneous

Use these only occasionally to make up your exchanges, as they contain a lot of fat, a lot of sugar, or are low in fibre.

1 cup of soup (tinned or packet)	2 sausages
2 level teaspoons Horlicks, Ovaltine	4 large chips
2 bun-size batter puddings	
1 small brickette (or scoop) ice cream	

† More detailed lists are available in Appendix 5.

†† Sliced bread varies according to the brand; the carbohydrate content will be found on the packaging. For further details of the carbohydrate content of these and other manufactured foods, you should refer to 'Countdown', published by the British Diabetic Association.

Which type of food should you choose?

Principles

Your food can be divided into three groups. To help you identify the group to which a particular food belongs, a colour coding system is used throughout this section:

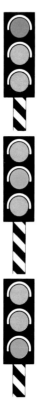

Food which you should try to avoid (except in cases of emergencies like hypo's or on special occasions) e.g. food containing large amounts of sugar.

Food which can be eaten with some care and regulated to a certain extent, e.g. refined starch carbohydrate (low in fibre) and full fat milk and milk products, and some fats.

Food which can be eaten regularly as part of the diet.

The diet you follow should enable you to maintain your weight without causing you to feel hungry. Such a diet will have to be worked out with you, in the first instance, by your doctor and/or dietitian, but some general guidelines are given below.

Foods to be eaten regularly	## Carbohydrate-containing foods

Carbohydrate and fibre

Recent evidence has indicated that the best choice from this group would be the wholegrain cereals, such as those found in wholemeal bread, wholemeal flour, and wholewheat breakfast cereals, for example Shredded Wheat, Puffed Wheat, Bran Flakes and All Bran (Fig. 3.16). It is thought that the presence of fibre in these foods reduces the rate of release of sugar into the blood after digestion, and of course this is much better for diabetic control.

You can select from Table 2 (see also Appendix 5) those carbohydrates with a high fibre content. These should provide up to two-thirds of your total carbohydrate requirements.

Fruit and vegetables

Fruit and vegetables (Fig. 3.16) should always be included in the daily diet. Not only are they a good source of carbohydrate, but they are also high in minerals and vitamins and many are high in fibre. Those that contain carbohydrate should be included in your total daily intake, as indicated in Table 2.

Foods which contain negligible amounts of carbohydrate

These are shown in Fig. 3.17 and listed in Table 3, page 46. A more detailed list is given in Appendix 5, Tables VII and XI. They include:

- Protein-containing foods, such as lean meat, fish, poultry and eggs †
- Fat-containing foods, but only low- or reduced-fat dairy products †
- Low-sugar beverages †
- Many vegetables and fruits.

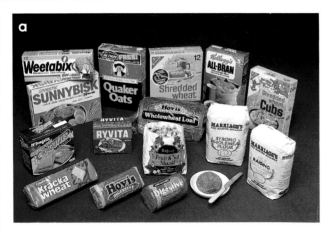

Fig. 3.16
The best choice of carbohydrate foods.

a. **Fibre-containing foods**

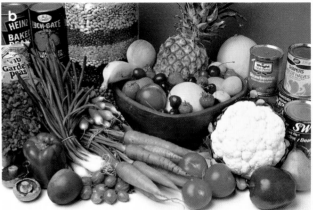

b. **Fruit and vegetables** (many of these contain fibre)

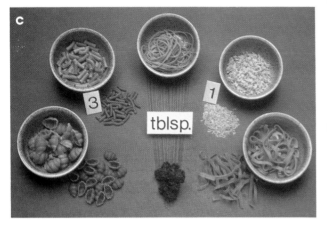

c. **Pasta and wholegrain rice**

Fig. 3.17
Foods which can be eaten regularly.

a. **Protein-containing foods** — care should be taken to limit the intake of fat.

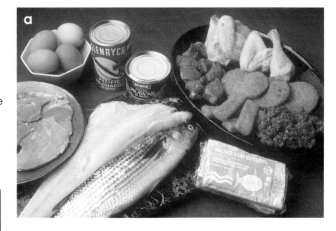

b. **Low-fat dairy products** — preferably, choose these in order to keep down the fat content of your diet. Milk or yoghurt will be part of your carbohydrate allowance.

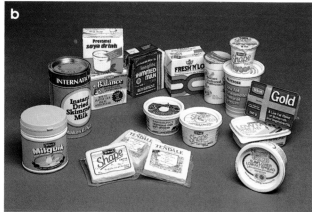

c. **Beverages** — sugar-free mixer drinks may be drunk freely.

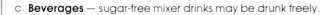

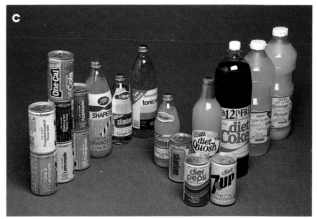

Proteins — meat, fish, poultry and eggs.

To have pleasant and nutritional meals, the balance of energy or calories is provided by protein (and fat). As Westerners, we eat considerably more protein than we really need, but luckily in normal amounts it does not affect the blood sugar.

Providing you take care to avoid a very fatty diet, by following the steps outlined on pages 49 and 50, meat, poultry, fish and eggs can be eaten.

Beverages

Drinks, listed in Table 4, page 52, contain no sugar. It should be remembered that milk in drinks, such as tea, coffee and cocoa, need to be counted with your exchanges.

TABLE 3 Foods which can be eaten freely

Vegetables

All green leafy vegetables, cauliflower, runner beans, carrots, peas, marrow, mushrooms, celery, onions, tomatoes, peppers, swede, turnip, broad beans, salad vegetables.

Fruit

Cranberries, gooseberries, lemons, loganberries, rhubarb, redcurrants, ½ grapefruit .

Beverages

Tea, coffee, Oxo, Bovril, Marmite, sugar-free diabetic squashes and 'mixers', soda water, tomato juice, lemon juice, clear soups.

Seasonings

Pepper, mustard, vinegar, pickles, herbs, spices, stock cubes, essences and food colourings.

Sweetening agents

Tablet and liquid saccharine sweeteners, aspartame and acesulfame-K.

Foods to be eaten with care and in regulated amounts

Carbohydrates

Foods in this group include rapidly absorbed carbohydrates, which are low in fibre and which lead to a more rapid rise in blood sugar. Ideally, they should be chosen to provide no more than a third of your exchanges. A typical selection is shown in Figs. 3.18 and 3.19.

Fig. 3.18
Foods to be eaten in regulated amounts.

a. **Bread:** whenever possible eat wholemeal bread, since white bread has had the fibre removed and may cause a more rapid rise in blood sugar.
Cereals: although they may be relatively low in sugar, if they are also without fibre, which slows down the absorption, they may produce a more rapid rise in blood sugar than a high fibre but sugar-containing cereal.
White flour products: e.g. crackers, should be eaten only if the general diet contains some fibre.

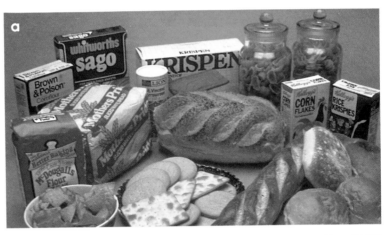

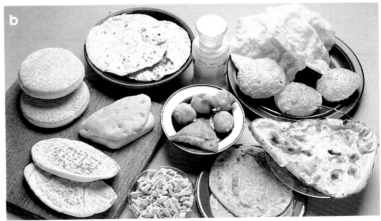

b. These Asian and West Indian foods are not only made with refined flour, but many also contain a lot of extra fat. Therefore, they are to be eaten with restraint, particularly when trying to lose weight.

Dairy Products

- **Milk** (Fig. 3.19) is a useful food to include every day, but does contain sugar (see Table 3, page 46) and should be considered as an exchange or portion.

- **Yoghurt** is a popular dairy product, but it is better to buy plain, unsweetened yoghurt and add a small helping of fruit, rather than to use sweetened fruit yoghurt.

Fig. 3.19.
Dairy products should be eaten in limited quantities.

- **Other milk products** (Fig. 3.19), such as evaporated milk, can be taken in small quantities, but sweetened dairy products, for instance condensed milk, must be avoided.

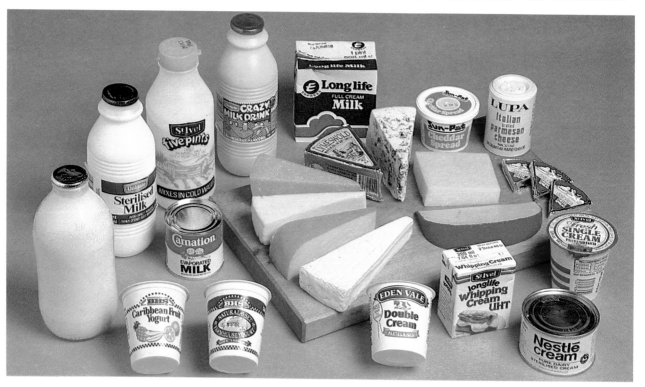

Foods to be eaten with caution

● **Fats** (Fig. 3.20) should be eaten with some restraint. They are a concentrated form of calories, which easily lead to

Fig. 3.20.
Foods to be eaten with caution.

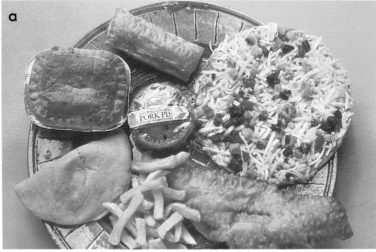

a. Many popular foods contain a high level of 'hidden' fat, particularly meat products, pastry and fried food such as fish and chips.

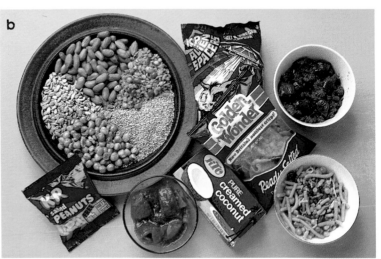

b. Other foods with a high 'hidden' fat content, include natural foods, such as nuts and seeds, and processed foods, such as crisps.

Fig. 3.20
c. All of these 'visible' fats should be limited.

overweight, and in excess may cause other health problems.

● **Meat Products** (Fig. 3.20a) which are particularly high in fat, such as sausages and meat pies, should be eaten in limited amounts. Also, you should remove the fat from meat.

● **Cheese, cream, butter and margarine** (Fig. 3.20c) should be limited. Do not nibble fatty foods.

Spread butter and other spreads sparingly. Try replacing milk with skimmed milk.

If you feel hungry and you are not overweight, it is likely that you need more carbohydrate. It is not necessary to base every meal on a large portion of meat, fish or cheese.

Ideal cooking methods are braising, stewing, dry roasting, grilling, baking in foil, poaching or scrambling. A useful maxim is: avoid the frying pan — grill instead.

Foods to be avoided

Avoid completely very sweet foods and drinks, which cause a rapid rise in blood sugar (Fig. 3.21). By cutting out sweet foods you are minimizing the amount of sugar which has to be disposed of by your reduced insulin supply. A detailed list of these is given in Table 4, page 52.

Fig. 3.21
A range of common foods which, because of their high sugar content, should be avoided.

a. Sweets and chocolates have a very high sugar content, especially fruit drops and pastilles.

b. These foods rapidly affect the blood sugar. Honey is often mistakenly believed to be suitable for those with diabetes.

c. Asian and West Indian sweetmeats, which are offered as part of hospitality and at festivals, should be eaten as 'small tastes' only.

d. Sweet biscuits and cakes should be substituted with plain, low sugar equivalents.

e. Instant desserts and sweetened cereals should be replaced with unsweetened alternatives.

f. These highly sweetened drinks should be avoided, unless you are hypoglycaemic.

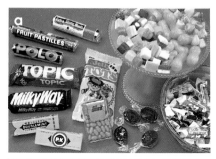

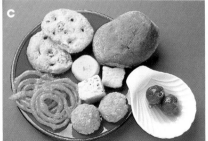

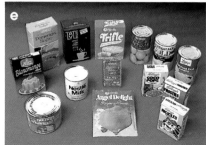

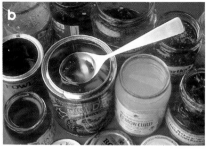

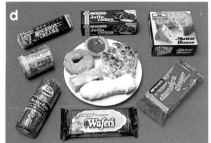

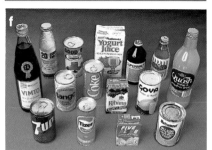

TABLE 4 Foods to be avoided

The foods listed below are high in sugar and have virtually no nutritional value. Therefore, they should not be eaten except during times of illness, or in emergencies, such as hypo's.

Marmalade*/jam*/honey*

Mincemeat/lemon curd

Golden syrup

Black treacle

Sugar

Glucose

Glucose tablets

Fizzy drinks*, cordials* and squashes*, unless marked 'no sugar' or 'low calorie'.

Minerals*

Coca Cola*

Lemonade*

Mixers such as ordinary tonic*, ginger ale* etc.

Bottled sauces and chutneys (in large amounts)

Buns

Pastries

Sweet biscuits

Fruit tinned in syrup*

*Low-sugar alternatives are available.

For further information refer to 'Countdown', published by the British Diabetic Association.

Diabetic foods

These are foods, usually sweet, in which cane sugar has been substituted with other sweeteners. They are best avoided, not only because they are very expensive, but because they are very often high in calories, and therefore fattening. Some specialist products, however, may add variety to the diet. These include the wide range of sugar-free drinks, fruits tinned in natural juices, and sugar-free sweets and chewing gum (Fig. 3.22).

Fig. 3.22
Good choices
Sugar-free and low-sugar drinks are suitable for those with diabetes.

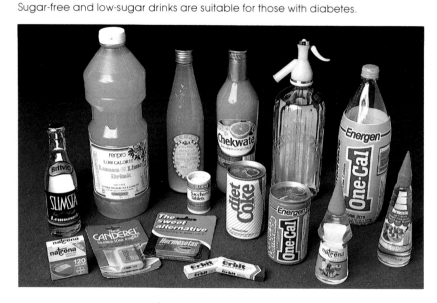

Sugar substitutes — which ones?

Saccharine, saccharine-based sweeteners, acesulfame-K or aspartame can be used by anyone with diabetes. Examples of these are the various tablet and liquid sweeteners, such as Hermesetas, Sweetex, Saxin, Natrena, Canderel, etc. (Fig. 3.22). Powder sweeteners, which are mixtures of saccharine and sugar, or saccharine and milk sugar, or saccharine and sorbitol, or fructose (fruit sugar) should not be used without individual advice from your dietitian, but they may be useful in baking or preserve making.

Alcohol

Alcohol need not be avoided, but some care should be exercised:

- Alcohol is a source of a considerable number of calories, which can cause significant weight problems (if you are overweight you should take advice from your doctor).
- Most beers, lagers and ciders are high in carbohydrate. Normally, one drink per day would be permitted as part of the calorie allowance.
- Particular care should be taken with beers described as 'low' in carbohydrate. They are not only expensive but have a higher alcohol and calories content than ordinary beers.
- Mixers, which contain sugar, should be avoided completely (see Table 4, page 52). Use 'slimline' varieties.
- Sweet wines are very variable in sugar content and are best avoided.
- Avoid liqueurs.
- Home-made wines and beers are very variable in both sugar and alcohol content.
- It is inadvisable to drink more than on average of three drinks daily on a regular basis and less is preferable — if you are needing to lose weight, a maximum of one a day.

  *NOTE: 1 drink is defined as ½ pint beer/lager OR 1 pub measure of spirits OR 1 small glass of sherry OR 1 glass of wine OR 1 pub measure of vermouth/aperitif.

Remember:

- **Never drink on an empty stomach**
- **Drink moderate quantities only**
- **Never drink and drive**

Eating out

As your knowledge about your diet increases, you will gain more confidence about eating out, and will be able to select from the menus those foods which are most appropriate. For those of normal weight, the modern diabetic diet is much less restrictive than diets recommended in the past.

Fig. 3.23.
Eating out.
With a little extra care you can eat out and still follow your diet.

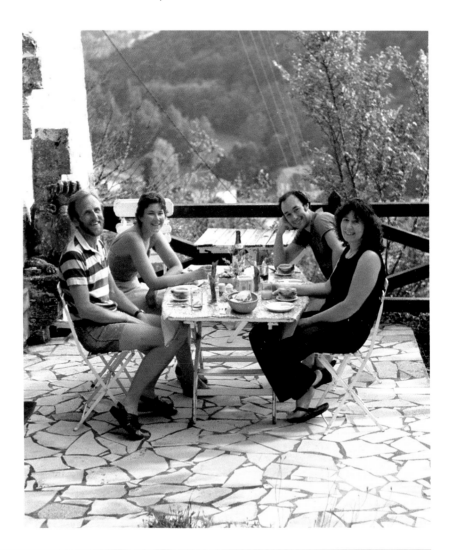

If you are at all concerned about the suitability of certain foods in a restaurant, do not be afraid to ask.

Wherever possible:

- Select generous portions of vegetables

- Cut down on fats and sugar

- Choose baked, grilled or boiled food, as opposed to fried or roasted.

However, an occasional indiscretion, although it may lead to a temporary rise in blood sugar, will not do any long-term harm.

Of course, eating with friends or relatives should pose no problems. If you let them know the foods you would prefer not to eat, any embarrassment will be readily avoided.

Losing weight when taking insulin

If you have diabetes and are overweight, losing weight will be highly beneficial to your health generally and particularly to your diabetes. It is likely that a reduction in weight will enable you to control your diabetes better.

However, if you are taking insulin, losing weight can be a problem, because dieting will undoubtedly upset the balance between your blood sugar levels and the insulin you inject. Therefore, if you decide to lose weight, your calorie and carbohydrate reduction will have to be planned carefully, with the help of your dietitian and doctor, otherwise hypoglycaemia can result.

If you need help

If you should have any problems with your diet, do not be afraid to ask for help from your doctor or dietitian. Very good guidance can be obtained from the many diabetic cookery books, and from the extensive lists of foods now available, such as 'Countdown', published by the British Diabetic Association.

Your family's diet

Although the type of diet outlined above is designed for the specific needs of a person with diabetes, it is a particularly healthy diet in so far as it is based on a minimal sugar and fat intake, and an increase in the consumption of fruit, vegetables and fibre-containing foods. Consequently, it is recommended that the whole family should be offered the benefits of meals based on this type of diet.

Fig. 3.24
Food for people with diabetes can be enjoyed by the whole family. Such food is not only healthier, but can be just as tasty as more conventional dishes.

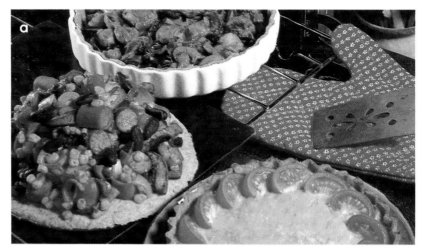

a. Frankfurter pizza, Mixed grill flan and Tuna flan.

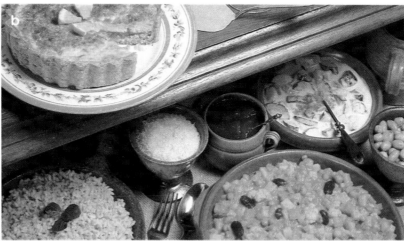

b. Cottage cheese quiche and Vegetable curry.

Fig. 3.25
Delicious sweets.
Strawberry water ice, Blackcurrant fool and
Mandarin surprise.

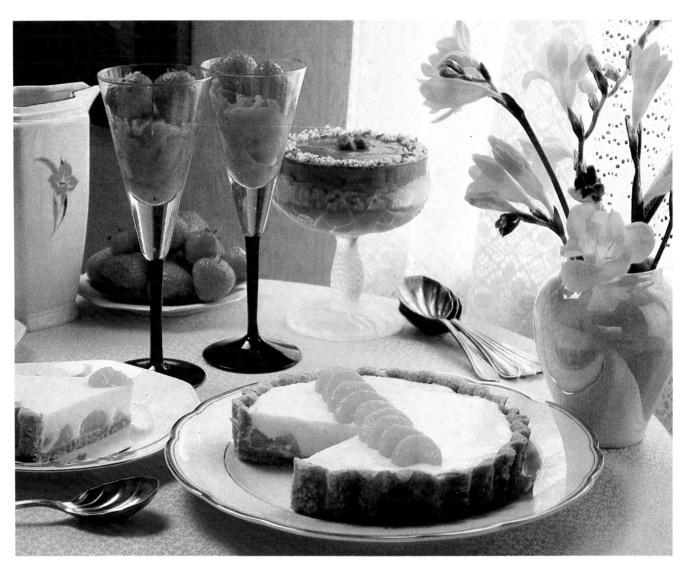

Summary

Your food can be divided into three groups.

Food which you should try to avoid (except in emergencies) e.g. food containing large amounts of sugar.

Food which can be eaten with some care and regulated to a certain extent, e.g. refined starch carbohydrate (low in fibre) and full-fat milk and milk products, and some fats.

Food which can be eaten regularly as part of the diet.

Planning your diet consists of the following steps:

- Determining the total number of carbohydrate portions per day
- Deciding when to have the portions
- Selecting the type of food suited to your taste
- Balancing meals and snacks with foods freely allowed, avoiding those containing too much sugar.

OTHER FACTORS AFFECTING CONTROL

We have discussed the two main elements of good diabetic control — insulin and diet — but three other important factors may alter the blood sugar level:

1. Exercise
2. Illness
3. Emotional stress.

Exercise

Whenever you take exercise or do physical work in any form, you burn up energy and lower your blood sugar. Thus, exercise and insulin work together to lower the blood sugar, and the more exercise you take, the less insulin you will need. This has been proved time and time again by those with diabetes who participate in sporting activities. For example, a well-known professional footballer found that while playing a first division game, he could keep his blood sugar normal with only a quarter of his usual insulin dose. Likewise, when involved in heavy manual labour, you will find that you will require less insulin on working days than when relaxing.

Clearly, exercise is beneficial to all people with diabetes, not only because it lowers blood sugar levels, but also because it makes the action of insulin on your fat and muscle cells more efficient.

However, if certain simple precautions are not taken, too much exercise, or exercise at the wrong time, can upset the balance of control. For instance, if you have taken insulin in the usual dose and are suddenly faced with unexpected exercise, this will cause an additional fall in blood sugar, which will have to be countered by an extra snack, in order to prevent the risk of hypoglycaemia (see Chapter 6, page 92). Alternatively, on days on which heavy exercise or work are anticipated, it may be necessary for you to reduce your insulin dose.

More information on types of exercise and diabetes is provided in the section on 'Exercise and sport', Chapter 9 page 123.

Fig. 3.26
Exercise is beneficial to all.
Whether you play sport, or you prefer less strenuous physical pursuits, like walking or gardening, exercise is good for you, because it burns up energy, lowers your blood sugar and makes the action of insulin more effective.

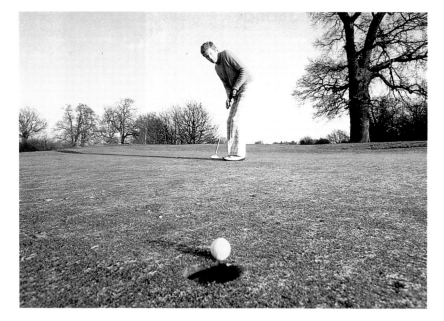

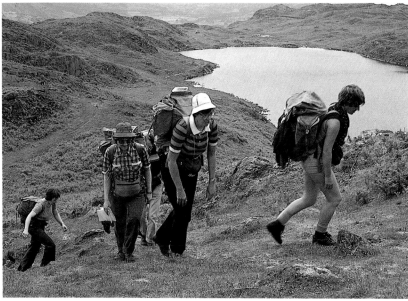

Photo: Dr Rowan Hillson

Illness and emotional stress

The chief effect of illness or stress is to increase the blood sugar, so that more insulin is then required. It is important that you understand the steps you need to take in order to return your blood sugar to normal, and these are considered in detail in the section 'What can go wrong?', Chapter 6, page 81.

Summary

Controlling your diabetes is a matter of reducing your blood sugar levels to normal, and then maintaining them within acceptable limits. In other words, you must restore the balance between 'sugar-in' and 'sugar-out'. There are four main elements affecting the blood sugar levels:

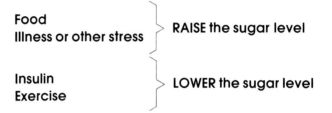

Food
Illness or other stress ⟩ **RAISE the sugar level**

Insulin
Exercise ⟩ **LOWER the sugar level**

Your blood sugar depends, therefore, on:
- What you eat
- When you eat
- Your dose of insulin
- The type of insulin
- Time of insulin injection
- The amount of exercise or physical work you take.

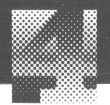

Is your treatment effective?

Why you need to carry out tests

The aim of treatment is to return your blood sugar level to as near normal as possible and to maintain it within acceptable limits. When you first start to treat your diabetes, you will want to be sure that the insulin doses and the amount and type of food you eat are appropriate — that the balance is right. Unfortunately, <u>how you feel is not an accurate guide to the level of your blood sugar,</u> since quite wide variations in blood sugar can occur without producing any symptoms. In fact, typical symptoms of diabetes — thirst, weight loss and the passing of large amounts of urine — appear only if your diabetes is badly out of control. Even with moderately high levels of blood sugar — the sort of levels which can, over a period of years, lead to serious complications — you may have no symptoms.

Therefore, it is essential that you are able to make some form of check on the blood sugar level, and that you are able to repeat these checks at frequent intervals. These tests are necessary for three reasons:

1. To help you to understand what produces high or low blood sugar levels — <u>this will enable you to make appropriate adjustments, in order to avoid a too high or a too low blood sugar level.</u>

2. To determine if your treatment is effective — <u>if it is not, you will be able to make any necessary changes in the type and dose of insulin, or in the size and timing of your meals.</u>

3. To reassure yourself that the best possible control is being achieved — <u>this will help to ensure your long-term health.</u>

Blood tests v. urine tests

The best way to determine the effects of food, insulin and exercise on blood sugar is indirectly by urine tests, or directly by blood tests.

Urine tests, are easy to perform, but have the disadvantage that they only tell you when the blood sugar has been too high and not when it is too low. Also, because they provide an indirect measurement, they are less informative than blood tests.

Blood tests, on the other hand, have significant advantages, not only in the early stages of insulin treatment, but also long-term, especially in those who have difficulty in maintaining control, or in those predisposed to disabling hypoglycaemic reactions. They give an exact reading of the blood sugar <u>at the time of testing.</u> Tests are now available which enable you to measure your own blood sugar levels accurately, while at home, work or wherever you might be.

Blood tests

Technique

Blood tests (Fig. 4.1) require you to obtain a drop of blood, which must then be allowed to react with a specially prepared testing strip, producing a change in colour.

Fig. 4.1
Blood tests
a. A drop of blood can be obtained by pricking the finger.

b. The Autolet® automatically pricks your finger after you push the release.

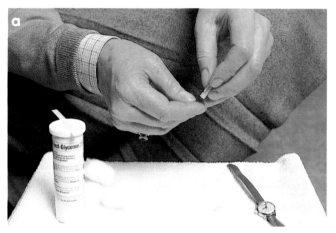

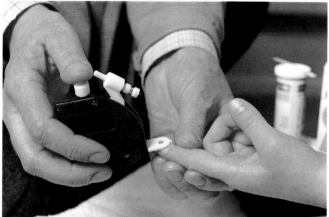

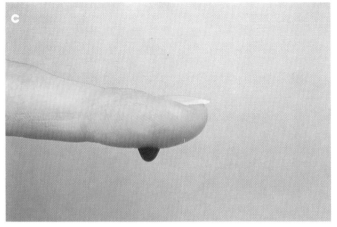

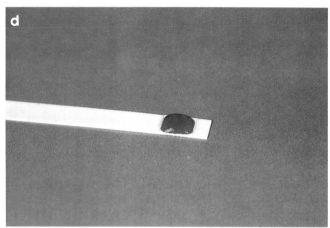

c. The drop of blood should be large enough to cover the test zones on the strip.

d. With the test strip held horizontally, apply the blood sample.

Depending on the test used, the blood sugar level is determined either by visually comparing the colour of the test strip against the colour scale provided (Fig. 4.2), or by using a special meter (Fig. 4.3). The results are then recorded (Fig. 4.4).

Fig. 4.2
Blood tests — determining the blood sugar level visually.

a. Visidex II

b. BM-Test Glycemie 20-800

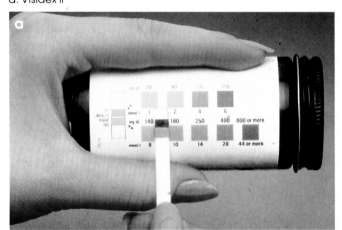

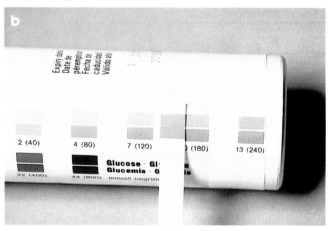

Fig. 4.3
Blood tests — determining the blood sugar level using a blood glucose monitor.

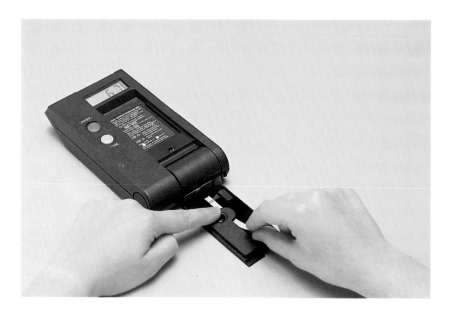

Fig. 4.4
Blood tests — recording the test results.
Always record your test results using a record diary such as this.

MONTH		TEST TIME							INSULIN		COMMENTS
Day	Date	Before B/Fast	After B/Fast	Before Lunch	After Lunch	Before Dinner	Evening	Before Bed	AM	PM	REACTIONS, MEDICATION, ILLNESS, ETC.
	1	10		7		4			28	14	
	2						10		28	14	
	3	2		4		7			28	14	
	4	7						7	28	14	
	5	7	2*						28		* Hypoglycaemic reaction at 12.30
	6										

Blood tests are simple to perform, and usually almost painless. Full details are provided in Appendex 3, page 197.

Interpreting the results and making adjustments

The blood sugar level rises after meals, and is at its lowest before meals; in people without diabetes this variation is kept within quite a narrow range. The accepted way of expressing blood sugar concentration is by millimoles per litre, and is written mmol/l, e.g. 8 mmol/l. The main points to remember are that the normal range of blood sugar before meals is between 4 and 10 mmol/l (Fig. 4.5), and when perfectly controlled does not exceed 10 mmol/l, even after meals.

Fig. 4.5
The normal range of blood sugar before and after meals.

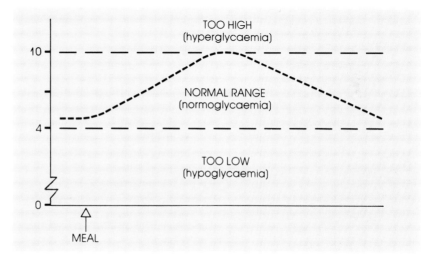

The aim of your treatment is to get your blood sugar as close as possible to this range. Your blood tests will help you to achieve this, but you must always interpret your tests with caution and not react hastily. For example, if your blood sugar is high <u>before</u> lunch you should not immediately jump to the conclusion that more insulin is necessary. Instead, you should think of the possible reasons for this unexpectedly high reading.

Possible explanations include:

- Having eaten too much during the morning
- Lack of exercise or less physical work than usual
- Worry or stress
- Not enough insulin
- A faulty reading.

If, on the other hand, the blood sugar is low before a meal, you should certainly consider having something to eat, and if it happens consistently, you should have less insulin (see also the section 'Hypoglycaemia', Chapter 6, page 85).

The adjustments you can make to your treatment are considered in more detail in Chapter 5, page 73.

How often should the blood be tested?

To start with you will be asked to perform tests several times a day, in order to help you understand what causes changes in your blood sugar. Once diabetic control is good, and if little variation in insulin dosage is required, tests may be made about once or twice a day. However, there are occasions when you may find it useful to carry out tests more often, e.g:

- If you are troubled by hypoglycaemia
- If your work, exercise or meal times vary a great deal
- During the week or two before a routine clinic visit, when more frequent tests will enable you and your doctor to discuss whether any changes in insulin treatment might be required.

When are blood tests essential?

There are three occasions when testing is essential:

1. If you feel unwell
2. If you suspect that your blood sugar is falling too low, and especially if you are about to drive or embark on something hazardous
3. If you are planning a pregnancy (see Chapter 8, page 110).

Urine tests

How urine tests work and their interpretation

The blood sugar can be measured indirectly by testing your urine. This is possible because as the blood sugar rises, there comes a point at which it starts to leak into the urine. This happens when the level of the blood sugar is too high, usually above about 10 mmol/l. Therefore, if the blood sugar has exceeded this threshold level since you last passed urine, a test for sugar in the urine will be <u>positive</u> (Fig. 4.6a), whereas if the blood sugar has not exceeded this level (normal) the urine test will be <u>negative</u> (Fig. 4.6b). If the test is positive, the amount of sugar present gives an approximate guide to how high the level in the blood has risen above the threshold. Thus, with your type of diabetes, most tests should be <u>negative.</u> But, remember, urine tests are of limited value only, because they do not tell you <u>when</u> the blood sugar is too low.

Fig. 4.6
How urine tests work.

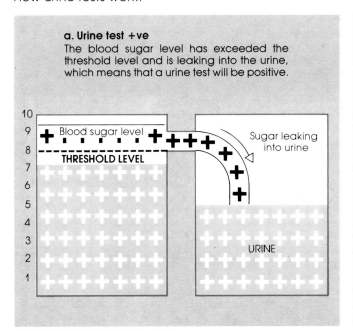

a. Urine test +ve
The blood sugar level has exceeded the threshold level and is leaking into the urine, which means that a urine test will be positive.

Blood sugar level

Sugar leaking into urine

THRESHOLD LEVEL

URINE

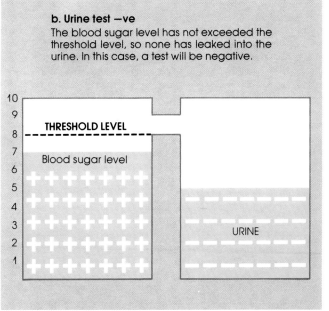

b. Urine test −ve
The blood sugar level has not exceeded the threshold level, so none has leaked into the urine. In this case, a test will be negative.

THRESHOLD LEVEL

Blood sugar level

URINE

Which urine tests?

Three tests (Fig. 4.7) are commonly available in the United Kingdom:

1. **Clinitest,** which involves adding a tablet to urine diluted in a test tube, and observing the change in colour.
2. **Diastix,** which involves placing a strip of special paper in the stream of urine, and then observing the colour change.
3. **Diabur-Test 5000,** used similarly to Diastix.

Fig. 4.7
Urine test kits.
a. Clinitest
b. Diastix
c. Diabur-Test 5000
d. Test record card

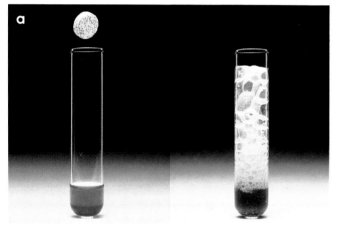

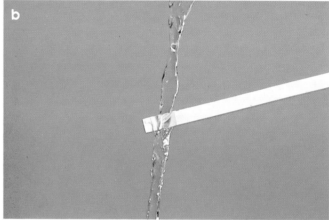

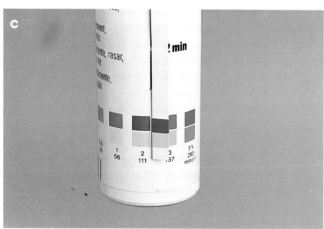

d Clinitest Record Chart

Report to Physician

Patient's Name_____ Doctor_____

Patient's Address_____
Perform test. Record date. Report results in appropriate column.

Date	Before Break-fast	Before Midday Meal	Before Evening Meal	Before Bedtime Snack	Other Information
Mar. 4	neg.		neg.	neg.	
5	neg.	neg.	++	neg.	
6	neg.	neg.	neg.	+ve	
7	trace		neg.	neg.	
8	neg.	neg.	neg.	neg.	
9	neg.		neg.	neg.	
10	++++				

All tests are satisfactory. Clinitest is easier to observe, but Diabur-Test 5000 and Diastix are simpler to use.

You will, of course, be shown how to test your urine when you first develop diabetes. For reference, full details of the three common tests are provided in Appendix 2, page 189. Urine tests depend on a colour change, so if you cannot see well, or you are colour blind, you may not be able to detect the change, and the tests may need to be done for you.

How often should you test?

To start with, you will be asked to test before each meal and last thing at night. This routine testing will help you to understand what increases your blood sugar — and hence turn your urine tests positive — and ensure that your insulin dose is correct. As your blood sugar returns to normal, and if all your urine tests become negative, only a few tests a week may be required, just to reassure you that all is well.

There are occasions, however, when you must test several times a day:

● If you feel unwell

● If you plan a pregnancy.

When should you test?

Ideally, all tests should be negative, but it is not always possible to achieve this. Testing before a meal is preferable; testing after a meal may produce positive results, since there is usually a small peak in the blood sugar immediately after eating.

Urine tests can be misleading

Urine tests can be misleading. For example some people are understandably perplexed when they feel hypoglycaemic, but their urine test is positive.

This occurs because some of the urine being tested may have been formed as much as one or two hours earlier, when the blood sugar was still high. Since that time, however, the blood sugar may have returned to a low level, but the earlier overspill of sugar from the blood (when the level was high), will still be registering in the urine and giving a positive result to your test. This problem may be overcome by emptying the bladder, waiting a short time (about half an hour), emptying the bladder a second time, and testing this urine specimen. This procedure, which is called 'double-voiding', produces a result which is more likely to relate to the blood sugar level at the time of testing.

Another reason for a false result is that some people leak sugar into the urine even when the blood sugar level is not increased — they have what is called 'a low renal threshold'. In such cases, testing will show the urine to be full of sugar, even though the blood sugar is normal. Clearly, to increase the insulin dose would merely cause the blood sugar to fall too low. This condition is rare, but if you think you have a low renal threshold you can check the situation by means of a blood test.

Testing for ketones

Ketones only appear when the blood sugar is very poorly controlled and you are unwell. Therefore, it is not necessary for you to test for ketones routinely, although this may be done if you are receiving treatment in hospital, or if you are prone to repeated illnesses.

Details on testing for ketones are given in Appendix 2, page 196.

A final comment

Whether blood or urine testing, <u>never</u> omit tests altogether, because without them you really have no idea what your control is like.

If you perform regular blood tests, it is not necessary to carry out urine tests as well.

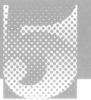

Keeping perfect balance

When should you make adjustments?

The aims of your treatment are to:

- Maintain your blood sugar within limits (i.e. blood tests between 4-10 mmol/l)

- Keep most of your urine tests free of sugar

- Ensure freedom from hypoglycaemia.

For some people with diabetes, however, these goals are not easy to achieve, because their way of life may vary considerably from one day to the next. Therefore, there may be a need for some variation in the amount of insulin injected, or in the type and amount of food eaten. As a guide, you should consider whether you need to change your insulin or food if:

- You are having frequent hypoglycaemic reactions

- You start to show sugar regularly in urine tests

- You are doing blood tests and they regularly show 10 mmol/l or more.

Two important points must be borne in mind, however, before making any changes to your insulin or food:

1 Never change your insulin dose on the basis of a single test, but only when repeated tests indicate a definite pattern.

2 A test tells you only how well the previous injection of insulin has worked — not the size of your next dose.

What type of adjustments might be necessary?

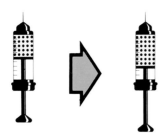

Various adjustments are possible:

- Changing your dose of insulin
- Changing the type of insulin and/or the balance between insulins
- Changing the timing of your insulin injection
- Changing the amount of food you eat
- A temporary change in insulin dosage
- Increasing the number of injections
- Altering your injection site.

Changing your dose of insulin

Depending on the results of your tests, you might find it necessary to modify your dose of insulin. For example:

- If all your tests, morning and evening, are high, you need more insulin.
- If all your morning tests are high and the remainder normal (Fig. 5.1), you may need more insulin in the evening. But, be careful — sometimes the blood sugar may fall very low during the night, then rise before breakfast, when the insulin level has dropped.

Fig. 5.1
High morning tests.
These results suggest the need for a larger dose of insulin in the evening.

	Blood								Urine			
	Before breakfast	2hrs after breakfast	Before mid-day meal	2hrs after mid-day meal	Before evening meal	2hrs after evening meal	Before bed	During night	Before breakfast	Before mid-day meal	Before evening meal	Before bed
	13	7			7		10		++	neg.	neg.	neg.
	15	4			7		7		++++	neg.	neg.	neg.
	17	4			7		4		++++	neg.	neg.	neg.

An increase in insulin may make this worse, and a change in the type of insulin is then needed.

● If you regularly work hardest on one particular day, then reducing the dose of insulin on that day of the week, or increasing it on all the other days, may give you better control.

Remember, bigger doses last longer. If your pre-supper test is high, a larger dose in the morning may correct it.

● If you have regular insulin reactions in the late morning, a reduction in the morning dose may be appropriate, likewise with the evening dose for evening reactions.

Changing the type of insulin and/or the balance between insulins

If all your mid-day tests are normal or slightly low (Fig. 5.2), but at 5-6 pm your tests are higher, then your insulin is acting quickly, but not lasting for long enough. Perhaps you need a mixture of quick and slow (clear and cloudy) insulins; or, if you are already taking such a mixture, an increase in the slow (cloudy) and a decrease in the quick (clear).

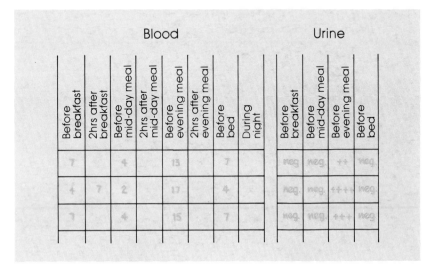

Fig. 5.2
High evening tests.
These results suggest the need for a change in the type and/or dose of insulin.

	Blood								Urine			
Before breakfast	2hrs after breakfast	Before mid-day meal	2hrs after mid-day meal	Before evening meal	2hrs after evening meal	Before bed	During night	Before breakfast	Before mid-day meal	Before evening meal	Before bed
7	4			13		7		neg.	neg.	++	neg.
4	7	2		17		4		neg.	neg.	+++	neg.
7		4		15		7		neg.	neg.	+++	neg.

If however your mid-day test is high and your pre-evening meal test normal (Fig. 5.3), perhaps more quick-acting clear insulin is needed in the morning.

Fig. 5.3
High mid-day tests and low evening tests.
These results suggest the need for more quick-acting clear insulin in the morning.

		Blood							Urine			
Before breakfast	2hrs after breakfast	Before mid-day meal	2hrs after mid-day meal	Before evening meal	2hrs after evening meal	Before bed	During night		Before breakfast	Before mid-day meal	Before evening meal	Before bed
4	15	15		7		7			neg.	++	neg.	neg.
7		15		7		4			neg.	++++	neg.	neg.
7		13		4		7			neg.	++++	neg.	neg.

Changing the timing of your insulin injections

Sometimes, increasing the interval between, say, your morning injection and breakfast, to a maximum of one hour, may give you better control of your blood sugar. Many may be unnecessarily concerned about the effects of delaying meals. If you take two injections a day, which permits a greater degree of flexibility than is available with one injection, any potential problems of delaying an evening meal or breakfast can be readily overcome:

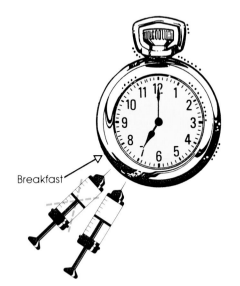

Breakfast

● **Late evening meal.** When you eat late, simply have a small snack at the time you would normally eat your evening meal (to balance any insulin that might be left over from your previous dose), then inject your insulin half an hour before your main meal.

If you intend eating an evening meal very much later than normal, then you should have slightly less insulin before your meal, otherwise the effects could continue into the next morning.

If in doubt about the time at which you will be eating, assume that the meal will be late and have a small snack in the meantime.

If you only have one injection a day, reverse the evening meal and bedtime snack, so that you have, say, a 20g (2 portions) snack at 6 pm and your main meal at 8.30 pm.

● **Late breakfast.** Occasionally, you may choose to have a lie-in and a late breakfast. This is perfectly acceptable, as long as you do not delay your breakfast by more than two hours, and you have your insulin half an hour before your late breakfast. You may need a cup of tea, or biscuit at your normal breakfast time, in case there is any insulin left over from the night before.

When working shifts, especially if the shifts change from day to day or week to week, it is often necessary to vary the time at which you inject your insulin. Certainly, the timing of injections will be different on working and rest days, and this, together with any variations in dosage, can be easily calculated by trial and error. Twice daily injections are usually essential.

Changing the amount of food you eat

The importance of taking extra carbohydrate to counter the effects of unexpected exercise and prevent hypoglycaemia have already been discussed on page 60. If you are normal weight and yet still hungry, or you are losing weight on the diet you have been given, there is no harm in increasing your portions, providing the increase is consistent from one day to the next. If, however, your tests begin to show high blood sugar levels, an increase in insulin dosage will easily correct this.

Another occasion when you may need to adjust your food intake, is when, for example, you feel slightly 'hypo', at around mid-day to 1pm (Fig. 5.4). An extra snack mid-morning, or an earlier mid-day meal often solves the problem, and may be easier than reducing your dose of insulin.

As a general rule, whenever your blood tests indicate that your blood sugar is too low, you should have more to eat, even if you feel well and do not feel particularly hungry.

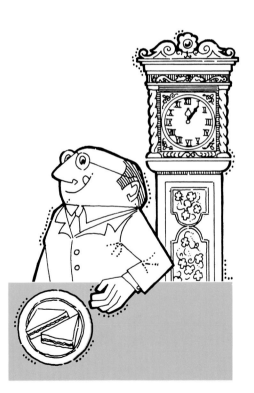

Fig. 5.4
Low mid-day tests.
These results suggest the need for a mid-morning snack or an earlier mid-day meal.

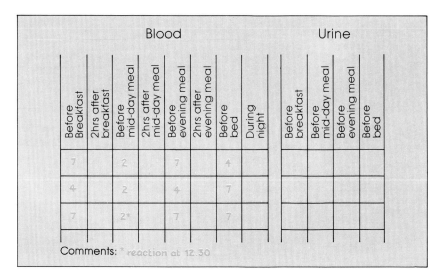

	Blood								Urine			
Before Breakfast	2hrs after breakfast	Before mid-day meal	2hrs after mid-day meal	Before evening meal	2hrs after evening meal	Before bed	During night		Before breakfast	Before mid-day meal	Before evening meal	Before bed
7	2			7		4						
4	2			4		7						
7	2*			7		7						

Comments: * reaction at 12.30

A temporary change in insulin dosage

The adjustments to your insulin dosage which are necessary when you are ill are described in Chapter 6, page 81. Often, you may find that minor ailments, such as a cold, cause your blood sugar level to rise for a few days. If you are a woman, you may find that a period causes an increase or decrease in your blood sugar level.

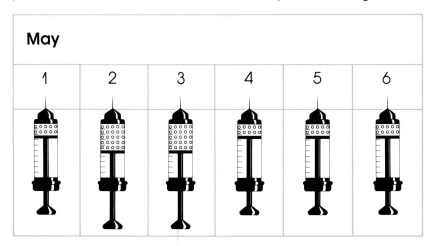

May

1	2	3	4	5	6

The commonest cause of fluctuations in the blood sugar is probably stress, and frequently you will find that the only indication that you are under pressure will be a raised blood sugar. Once you have made sure that this 'high' is not one isolated result, you should always respond to it by increasing your insulin, and then reducing it when the tests return to normal.

Increasing the number of injections

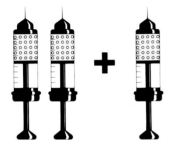

You may find it easier sometimes to take extra injections of quick-acting insulin, especially when having difficulties with control. For example, during an illness, when all your tests are high, an extra mid-day injection of insulin may control the situation (see page 84). If you have a very varied routine, you may find it easier to have a smaller injection of quick-acting insulin before each meal. Occasionally, an extra injection just before going to bed may help if difficulties are encountered early in the morning. Many variations are possible, enabling the correct balance to be achieved, even in the most varied of lifestyles.

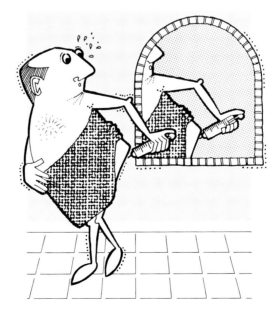

Altering your injection site

You may find that some variation in absorption of insulin and in control occur when injecting in different sites. Therefore, try to maintain consistency about where you inject (see Appendix 1, page 181).

Some final comments on adjustments

It is impossible in this Handbook to be specific about the exact changes you might need to make, because your diabetes is unique to you. In general, very small changes are likely to be of little benefit, and most err by changing too little rather than too much. If you are unhappy about making changes yourself, then seek advice. In time, your confidence will increase and you will get to know what changes to make, and when to make them.

You may find that you are able to maintain a very good balance with virtually no changes in insulin dosage or in the size of meals, from one day to the next. If you do have to make changes, however, try not to alter too many things too often and, having made a change, always wait for two or three days to see what happens, before making further alterations.

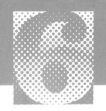

What can go wrong?

In this chapter we look at two important problems which can develop during treatment of your diabetes, and consider how to overcome them:

1 An <u>increase</u> in your blood sugar due to other illnesses — this can cause some resistance to the action of insulin, and ketosis.

2 Hypoglycaemia (a 'hypo' or 'reaction') — a blood sugar level which is <u>too low</u>, due to an imbalance between food and insulin.

It is **ESSENTIAL** that you are **PREPARED** for these problems and that you are able to deal with them. Therefore, it is important that you read and become familiar with this section of the Handbook.

KETOSIS OR SEVERE LACK OF INSULIN

Avoiding ketosis or severe lack of insulin

When is severe lack of insulin likely to occur?

It is most likely to happen:

- If the dose of insulin is reduced or not given at all
- In the presence of illness, which increases blood sugar and ketones by causing resistance to the action of insulin.

You may think because you feel unwell and do not want to eat, that you should reduce or even stop your insulin. This is a passport to disaster! In the absence of sufficient insulin your body breaks down fat as an alternative supply of fuel, and this is accompanied by the production of ketones. Eventually, if untreated, you would gradually develop a diabetic coma (ketosis). <u>This will not occur, however, if you are eating and drinking normally.</u>

Fortunately, symptoms develop relatively slowly (as compared with those of hypoglycaemia). Diabetic coma will be preceded by a period of <u>at least several hours</u> during which time the following symptoms may occur:

● A period of thirst
● Frequent passage of urine
● Weakness
● Vomiting.

What should you do if you are unwell?

To deal effectively with your diabetes during an illness, you must **BE PREPARED.** It is unlikely that you will feel like reading this Handbook when you are unwell, so get the following steps clear in your mind beforehand.

If you lose your appetite, feel sick or are vomiting, you should take the following steps:

STEP 1 — take fluids

You should try to have the equivalent of your normal intake or 'portions' of carbohydrates, but in the form of fluids. The reason for this is that fluids are absorbed from the stomach in considerable amounts, even if they are only kept down for a short while, and this will help to prevent the production of ketone acids. Therefore, you should substitute your portions with drinks, such as Lucozade and sweetened fruit juices, taking a glassful at hourly intervals. A list of fluid foods suitable to take when ill is given in Table 5.

STEP 2 — test your urine or blood

When you start feeling ill you should test your urine or blood, and continue to do so at least twice — and preferably four times — a day, or even more often. Unfortunately, when you are ill you will probably not feel like doing these tests, but it is during any illness that the results of such tests are particularly important, since your blood sugar may be rising and your dose of insulin may need adjusting.

TABLE 5 Foods/fluids to substitute for portions when off your food

<u>Fluids to provide 10g carbohydrate</u>
<u>(i.e. 1 Exchange/Portion/Line)</u>

Lucozade, or similar glucose drink	50ml/2fl oz
Grape juice (natural, bottled)	50ml/2fl oz
Fruit juices (natural, unsweetened), 1 wine glass	100ml/4fl oz
Coke or Pepsi, 1 wine glass	100ml/4 fl oz
Lemonade, or similar carbonated drink	150ml/5fl oz
Milk, 1 cup	200ml/7fl oz
Soup (thickened creamed, e.g. chicken), 1 cup	200ml/7fl oz
Soup (tomato tinned), ½ cup	100ml/4fl oz

<u>Foods to provide 10g carbohydrate</u>
<u>i.e. 1 Exchange/Portion/Line</u>

Ice-cream (plain), 1 scoop or small brickette	50g/2oz
Natural yoghurt, 1 pot	150g/5oz
Complan	3 level tablespoonsful
Drinking chocolate, Ovaltine, Horlicks or similar malted drink	2 heaped teaspoonsful
Sugar or glucose	2 level teaspoonsful
Honey, jam or syrup	2 level teaspoonsful
Oster rusks (Glaxo Farley)	2 rusks
Glucose tablets	3 tablets

<u>Other useful carbohydrate-containing foods</u>

	Carbohydrate content
Build-up (Carnation), 1 envelope	25g
Slender (Carnation), 1 envelope	20g
Sweetened fruit yoghurts, 1 pot (150g/5fl oz)	25-30g

STEP 3 — adjust your insulin dose

- **NEVER STOP TAKING INSULIN,** however ill you feel, or however little you are eating. The point to remember is that, even if you stop eating and continue to take your usual dose of insulin, <u>you will not become hypoglycaemic when you are ill</u>, because the body will automatically provide sugar from its stores.

- If the urine tests are negative, or the blood sugar less than 10mmol/l, continue with your usual insulin dose.

- If the urine tests show 1 to 2% of glycosuria, or the blood sugar is greater than 12 mmol/l, then your insulin dose should be increased. As a general rule, those on twice-daily clear (quick-acting) insulin should increase each dose by 4 to 8 units for as long as there is 1 to 2% glycorusia. This is a safe increase and will usually control the situation, although a greater increase may be required occasionally.

- If after about four hours you are still feeling or being sick, and your urine has become or is still full of sugar, or your blood sugar is greater than 12 mmol/l, you can take some more clear insulin.

- For those on a single daily injection of cloudy insulin, an increase of 8 to 12 units may be necessary. However, if the illness continues for more than a few hours, a switch to a twice-daily clear insulin will be necessary, and you will therefore need to consult your doctor. The actual amount by which you should increase your insulin dosage, should be determined by discussion with your doctor <u>before</u> you are ill.

- If, after a few hours, you are still vomiting, or have become very thirsty, and your tests are high, you need expert advice and should seek medical help.

HYPOGLYCAEMIA

When the balance is wrong

Good diabetic control rests on establishing, and then maintaining, a balance between meals taken at regular intervals and your injections of insulin (Fig. 6.1a).

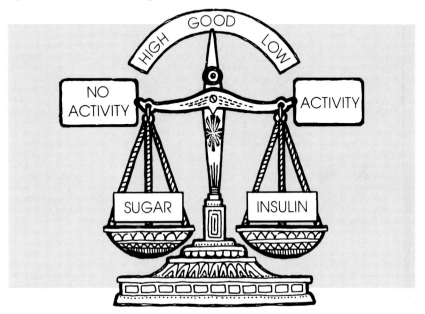

On occasions, such as when you have an unusually small meal (Fig. 6.1b), or you take unexpected exercise (Fig. 6.1c), or you forget your between meals snack (Fig. 6.1d) you may get this balance wrong, so that there is too much insulin relative to the amount of blood sugar. As a result, your blood sugar will fall too low and, unless this is rapidly treated, you may become unconscious. Therefore, it is important that you are able to:

● Recognize when this is occurring

● Take steps to put it right

● Prevent it from happening.

Fig. 6.1
Good diabetic control is a matter of balance.

a. The ideal balance between insulin and blood sugar occurs only with regular meals and regular insulin injections.

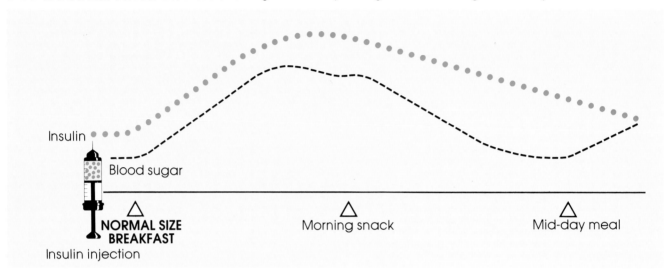

b. Poor balance can occur after an unusually small meal.

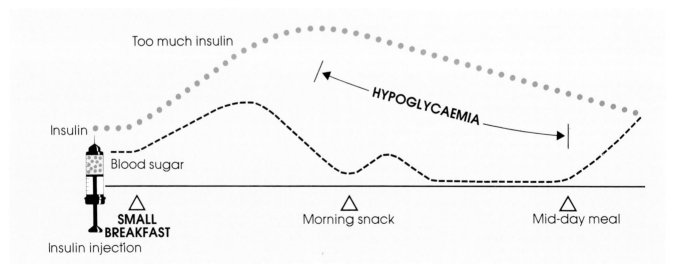

c. Unexpected exercise rapidly depletes the blood sugar, causing an imbalance.

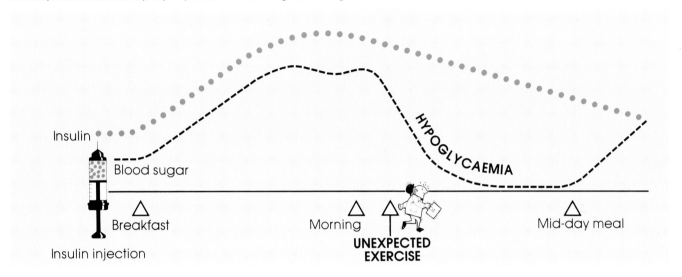

d. Forgetting a between-meals snack is a common cause of a reduced blood sugar level.

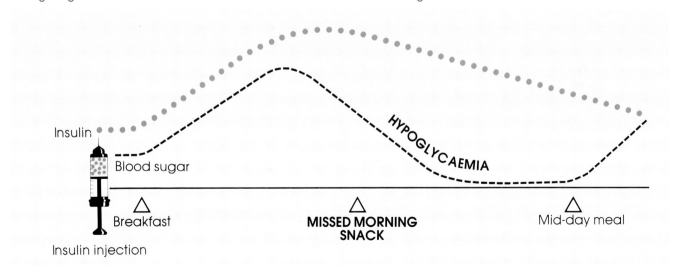

Recognizing hypoglycaemia

The common symptoms of hypoglycaemia include:
- Trembling
- Sweating
- Tingling around the mouth
- Palpitations of the heart, and then:
  Difficulty in concentration
  Confusion
  Muzziness
  Faintness
  Headache
  Blurring of vision
  Unsteadiness
  Irritability, bad temper
  Unusual lack of co-operation
  Vomiting may occur in children.

If the correct steps are not taken, these symptoms may be followed by:
- Loss of consciousness

- Convulsions (occasionally).

You will usually experience one or more symptoms, and these same symptoms will usually occur each time your blood sugar becomes too low.

If hypoglycaemia occurs at night, the early symptoms will usually wake you up. Occasionally, however, the only sign that your sugar has been low during the night may be a headache on waking in the morning.

But what happens if you fail to notice the initial symptoms during the night, and you therefore go into a hypoglycaemic coma? Fortunately, your body will eventually recognize what has happened, and will start to make sufficient sugar to bring about recovery. Death or disability does not occur as a result of hypoglycaemia, except when very large over-doses of insulin are given.

Treatment of hypoglycaemia

Immediate treatment will rapidly restore you to normal. It is important that, **AS SOON AS THE WARNING SYMPTOMS OCCUR,** you:

- **STOP** what you are doing. This is especially important if you are doing something which might involve risk to yourself or others, such as using machinery or driving.
- **IMMEDIATELY** take two lumps of sugar, or two teaspoonfuls of sugar in squash, or a glass of milk, together with a couple of biscuits (the amount needed is usually 1-2 exchanges). Within a few minutes the symptoms should have disappeared, but if not, take 2 more exchanges/portions (a list of suitable drinks and foods is given in Table 6).

TABLE 6 Foods/fluids which may be used to treat hypoglycaemia

	Amount providing 10g carbohydrate i.e. 1 exchange/portion/line
Lucozade, or similar glucose drink	50ml/2fl oz
Grape juice (natural bottled)	50ml/2fl oz
Fruit juices (natural unsweetened), 1 wine glass	100ml/4fl oz
Coke or Pepsi, 1 wine glass	100ml/4fl oz
Lemonade, or similar carbonated drink	150ml/5fl oz
Milk, 1 cup	200ml/7fl oz
Ice-cream (plain), 1 scoop or small brickette	50g/2oz
Natural yoghurt, 1 pot	150g/5oz
Complan	3 level tablespoonful
Drinking chocolate, Ovaltine, Horlicks or similar malted drink	2 heaped teaspoonful
Sugar or glucose	2 level teaspoonful/or 2 lumps
Honey, jam or syrup	2 level teaspoonful
Glucose tablets	3 tablets

Three essential precautions

1 **ALWAYS** carry some form of sugar which can be swallowed easily, as soon as you experience any symptoms of hypoglycaemia.

2 **ALWAYS** carry some identification that you have diabetes treated with insulin (Fig. 6.2). If you should fail to experience any symptoms, or you are unable to take some sugar or starchy food, you could become unconscious. It is essential that anybody who discovers you, should recognize that you have diabetes. Therefore, carry a card, such as the Dose Card produced by the British Diabetic Association, which provides clear instructions about the action that should be taken.

3 **ALWAYS** inform those who might need to know, such as workmates, relatives, teachers, etc., that there is a possibility that you could become hypoglycaemic.

Fig. 6.2
Always carry some form of identification.

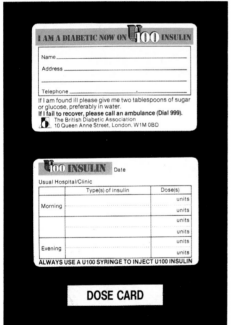

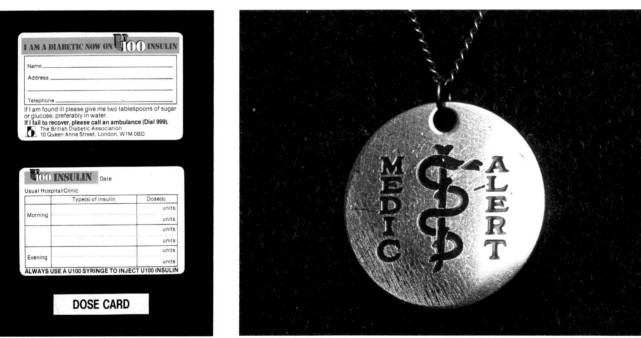

Advice to give your companions

It is important that your relatives, friends and work colleagues should recognize when you are suffering from hypoglycaemia, particularly if you are unaware of it and not taking the right steps. They should be instructed to take the following action:

● Stop you from continuing with any potentially dangerous activity.

● Persuade you to take some sugar, biscuits or a sweet drink, such as Lucozade or Ribena.

● If this is unsuccessful and you become incoherent or confused, they should try putting Dextrosol, or spooning sweetened fluid, into your mouth (not when you are lying down, though, since there is a risk that you might choke).

● If you should become unconscious, they **MUST NOT** try to give you sugar by mouth, but call a doctor, or take you to hospital immediately.

● Alternatively, they may give glucagon, but this is only necessary if you are subject to unexpected attacks of hypoglycaemia which cause unconsciousness. Glucagon is a hormone which, within a few minutes of being injected, will restore your blood sugar to normal, so that you will rapidly regain consciousness.

Your relatives, and perhaps a work colleague, should be taught the simple and safe technique of giving this injection (full details of glucagon injections are given in Appendix 4, page 201). As soon as you regain consciousness, you <u>must</u> take some food or sugar, because the effect of glucagon is only temporary.

Preventing hypoglycaemia

You should avoid hypoglycaemic reactions, not only because they are unpleasant and can prove embarrassing, but also because they could be dangerous if, for example, you are driving, or operating machinery.

Hypoglycaemic reactions will occur when there is no longer a balance between your blood sugar and the insulin you inject. The commonest times are:

- Mid-morning or before lunch

- During the night

- After exercise.

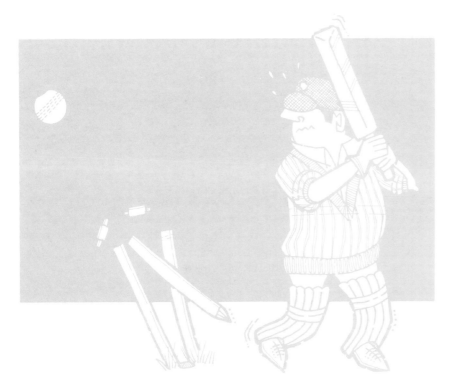

Exercise and hypoglycaemia

How can exercise cause hypoglycaemia?

When you take exercise, your muscles use up more sugar at a more rapid rate than when your muscles are at rest. Thus, because exercise can rapidly lower the blood sugar, there is a tendency to develop hypoglycaemic reactions (see Fig. 6.1c). These can be prevented, however, by following either of two courses of action:

- Taking extra carbohydrate

- Reducing your insulin dosage.

Taking extra carbohydrate

If you take any form of exercise, you will quickly learn how much extra carbohydrate you require for that particular activity. As a general guideline, it is recommended that 10-20g (1-2 portions) of rapidly absorbed carbohydrate, such as a couple of sweet biscuits, a Mars bar, or lumps of sugar, should be taken before any unusual activity. If the activity is prolonged or very strenuous, a further 10-20g of more slowly absorbed starch, such as bread or digestive biscuits, should be eaten, followed by another 10-20g after a couple of hours. The effect of exercise may be prolonged, which explains why, sometimes, even though extra carbohydrate may have been taken before and after exercise, a person with diabetes may still become hypoglycaemic several hours later.

Performing regular blood tests will help you to determine at which time you are most likely to be hypoglycaemic, and thus at which time of the day preventive action should be taken.

Reducing your insulin dosage

Reducing the insulin dosage is preferable treatment in cases when you know that extra exercise or strenuous work is expected. For example, regular daily work, Monday to Friday, involving steady physical exertion, such as bricklaying or gardening, can be best coped with by reducing the insulin on working days, with perhaps higher doses during the less active weekends. This will have to be combined with extra carbohydrate in the case of very strenuous activity.

The sedentary worker, however, should take normal doses of insulin during the week and if, say, he is an active gardener, then the dose of insulin might be reduced at the weekend.

At weekends, or when children return to school after the holidays, a reduction in insulin dosage may be helpful.

Some final comments

To prevent reactions, the aim must be to maintain the balance. Therefore, make sure that you:

 DON'T miss meals or snacks.

 DON'T delay your meals, especially the mid-day meal.

 DON'T skimp on your meals, but make sure that you are eating sufficient food.

 DON'T take too much heavy exercise without increasing your carbohydrate intake or reducing your insulin dose.

If, having checked that none of the above apply, you still have frequent reactions, an increase in your portions, or a reduction in insulin dose, may be necessary. Remember:

- CLEAR insulin reaches its maximum 4-5 hours after an injection, i.e. mid-day after a 7.30 a.m. injection, or midnight after an evening injection.

- CLOUDY insulin reaches its maximum 6-10 hours after an injection, i.e. mid-afternoon, or in the early hours of the morning.

A word of warning

Although the aim is to prevent hypoglycaemia, you must not achieve this by running a constantly high blood sugar. A high blood sugar may ensure against hypoglycaemic reactions, but over a prolonged period it will cause serious and permanent damage.

Long-term complications

After many years of diabetes, some of the body's tissues may be damaged, particularly the nerves of the feet, the eyes and the kidneys. However, many people are spared these problems, and there are those who, even after more than forty years of diabetes, show no trace of any diabetic complications.

Damage to the feet

Long-term diabetes sometimes results in nerve damage (called neuritis or neuropathy), which mainly affects the sensation in the feet. The hazard of this condition is that the majority of those in whom it occurs are not aware of the subtle decrease of sensation in their feet.

The feet normally undergo a lot of wear and tear, and any injuries are usually noticed because of discomfort. If, however, these are not felt, because of neuritis, increasing damage may pass unnoticed. In addition, any damage may be aggravated by diminished circulation. Ulceration and infection which then occur, can be very serious and result in prolonged periods off work, in bed, or in hospital, and sometimes require operations or even amputations. However, these injuries can, to a large extent, be avoided if proper care is taken of the feet. Therefore, the 'do's' and 'don'ts' of foot care are of great importance, and you should read the following section carefully.

Prevention of foot problems

Scrupulous attention to the care of the feet can prevent serious complications. The following measures and precautions are **ESSENTIAL.**

Inspecting your feet

● Inspect your feet regularly — ideally, daily — and if you cannot do this yourself, ask a friend to do it for you. This inspection is important because you may not always be able to feel bruises or sores.

● Seek advice if you develop any cracks or breaks in the skin, any calluses or corns, or your feet are swollen or throbbing. Advice from a State Registered Chiropodist is freely available under the N.H.S.

Washing your feet

● Wash your feet daily in warm water.

● Use a mild type of toilet soap.

● Rinse the skin well after washing. Dry your feet carefully, blotting between the toes with a soft towel.

● Dust with plain talc and wipe off any excess, so that it does not clog between the toes.

● If your skin is too dry, wipe your feet with lanolin, or an emulsifying ointment. This should be gently rubbed in after bathing your feet.

● If your skin is too moist, wipe your feet over with surgical spirit, especially between the toes. When the spirit has dried, dust the skin with talcum powder or baby powder.

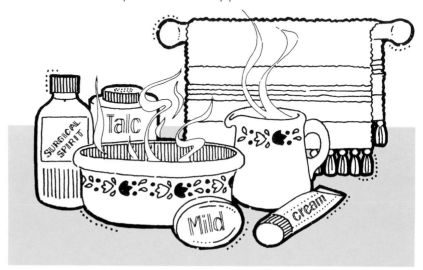

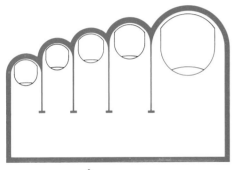

Nail cutting

- When the toenails need cutting, do this after bathing, when the nails are soft and pliable. Do not cut them too short.
- Never cut the corners of your nails too far back at the sides, but allow the cut to follow the natural line of the end of the toe.
- Never use a sharp instrument to clean under your nails or in the nail grooves at the sides of the nails.
- If your toe nails are painful, or if you experience difficulty in cutting them, consult your chiropodist.

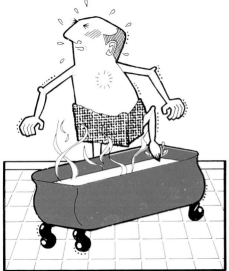

Heat and cold

- Be careful to avoid baths which are too hot.
- Do not sit too close to heaters or fires.
- Before getting into bed, remove hot water bottles, unless they are fabric covered. Electric under-blankets should be switched off or unplugged.
- If your feet get wet, dry them, and put on dry socks as soon as possible.
- Do not use hot fomentations or poultices.

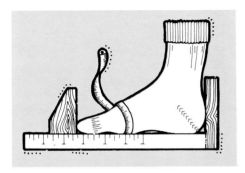

Shoes

Shoes must fit properly and provide adequate support. In fact, careful fitting and choice of shoes is probably the most important measure you can take to prevent diabetic foot problems. Therefore:

- Wear good fitting shoes. They <u>must</u> be comfortable.
- Never accept shoes that have to be 'broken-in' before being comfortable.
- When buying new shoes, always try them on, and rely on the advice of a qualified shoe fitter. Shoes must always be the correct shape for your feet.

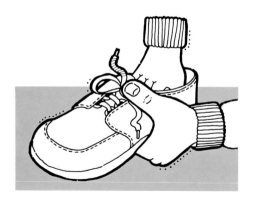

- Slippers do not provide adequate support and therefore should be worn only for short periods, night and morning, and not throughout the day. Do not walk about in bare feet.
- Do not wear garters.
- Make it a daily rule to feel inside your shoes for stones, nails etc.
- As you get older, avoid walking barefoot.

Corns and calluses

- Do not cut your corns and calluses yourself, or let a well-meaning friend cut them for you.
- Do not use corn paints or corn plasters. They contain acids which can be extremely dangerous to a diabetic.

First aid measures

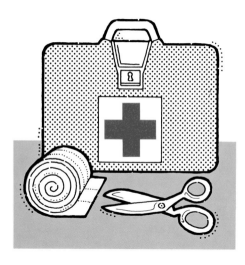

- Minor injuries, such as cuts and abrasions, can be self-treated quite adequately, by gently cleaning the area with soap and water and covering it with a sterile dressing.
- If blisters occur, do not prick them. If they burst, dress them as for a minor cut.
- Never use strong medicaments, such as iodine, Dettol, Germaline or other powerful antiseptics.
- Never place adhesive strapping directly over a wound.
- If you are in the slightest doubt about how to deal with any wound, discolouration, corns, and especially ulcers, consult your doctor.

Damage to the eyes

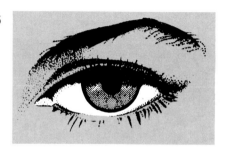

Two parts of the eye are affected by diabetes:

1. **The lens**

   Opacities in the lens (cataracts) are common in elderly people, and sometimes cause deterioration of vision. Cataracts are more common in people with diabetes.

2. The retina

This is the sensitive part of the back of the eye, which is responsible for transmitting visual images to the brain. Diabetes quite often causes minor abnormalities of the retina, without causing deterioration of vision — a condition described by the term 'diabetic retinopathy'. This takes several years to develop, and is extremely rare in children. In a minority of sufferers, however, vision does deteriorate, and in a few the affected eye becomes blind, usually from bleeding (haemorrhage) within the eye.

Prevention and treatment of eye damage

When cataracts seriously interfere with vision, they may be treated by operation.

Fortunately, damage to the retina can now be treated and blindness prevented in many instances. Treatment is by laser, a process which involves aiming a fine beam of very bright light at the diseased blood vessels. It is very simple to perform and is often successful, but it has to be undertaken before sight has deteriorated too seriously.

Therefore, it is essential that you should have your eyes tested and the backs of your eyes examined regularly — ideally, annually. This can be done by an optician, by doctors in the diabetic clinic, or by an eye specialist.

Some blurring of vision may occur in the first few weeks of treatment, but this is of no consequence and nearly always resolves within a week or two — so don't get your glasses changed. Subsequently, if you should notice a sudden loss of vision in either eye, you must report to your doctor immediately.

Painful neuritis

Sometimes — in fact, rather rarely — diabetic neuritis causes pain, usually in the feet and legs, which is particularly disagreeable. A burning sensation, a feeling of pins - and - needles, with an excruciating discomfort on contact with clothes or bedclothes, are the main characteristics of this condition. Unpleasant though most of these symptoms are, they almost always disappear in time, although it may take many months for them to do so. Very good diabetic control is essential. Various tablets, including pain-killers, are also used in its treatment.

Impotence

Sometimes, though probably not very often, nerve damage causes impotence. It should be remembered, however, that impotence is also common in those without diabetes. It is often due to psychological causes, and for this reason it is sometimes difficult to discover whether or not it is due to the nerve damage resulting from diabetes. Proper diagnosis is important, and specialist advice should be sought from your doctor or from trained counsellors (whose addresses can be found either from a general practitioner or from family planning clinics). Treatment is very difficult and not always successful.

Damage to the kidneys

Damage to the kidneys occurs less frequently than eye damage. Damage must be present for many years before function begins to deteriorate, and even then a few more years usually elapse before the situation becomes serious. Unfortunately, kidney disease does not give rise to symptoms until it is quite advanced. Therefore, early detection by means of regular checks from your doctor are very important.

Arterial disease

Degeneration or hardening and narrowing of the arteries (blood vessels) are normal consequences of ageing, but with diabetes there may be slight acceleration of this process. Arterial disease can result in heart attacks, and cause poor circulation in the feet and legs.

Treatment of arterial disease is exactly the same as those without diabetes. You should take the following precautions:

- Don't smoke
- Have your blood pressure checked yearly and treated if necessary
- Avoid too much fat in the diet, and do not become overweight
- Take as much exercise as you can and you will keep these risks to the minimum.

LONG-TERM COMPLICATIONS — POINTS TO REMEMBER

The following points must be emphasized:

- The problems of long-term diabetes occur only in a minority.
- Good control of diabetes often prevents the development of these complications.
- Smoking accelerates arterial disease (affecting heart and feet) and should be avoided.
- Obesity is often associated with arterial disease. Therefore, you should try to control your weight by an approved diet and exercise.
- Regular clinic attendance will ensure the early detection and treatment of any complications.

Clinic attendance

The organization of clinics

Your local diabetic clinic plays an important role in the treatment and control of your diabetes. The organization of these clinics varies in different areas of the country. In the majority of cases it is at the local hospital and is under the direction of a hospital consultant. In some areas, however, clinics have been set up in specially trained general practices, or co-operative schemes have been developed between hospital specialists and general practitioners. Evening clinics may be held to enable you to attend after work.

Fig. 7.1
Regular visits to your diabetic clinic are essential.

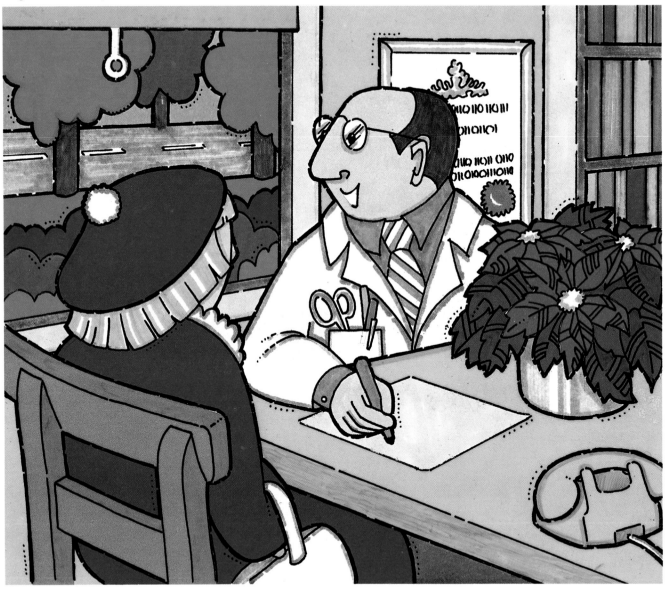

When is it necessary to attend the clinic?

If your diabetes has been diagnosed only recently, you will need to attend the clinic quite regularly, possibly every few weeks. When you understand your diabetes and when you have achieved satisfactory control, your clinic attendance may be less frequent, perhaps once every few months, with a yearly check on your general health.

If your control is good and you have no problems, you may think it a waste of time to attend the clinic. This is not the case, however, and there are a number of very good reasons why it is essential that you attend the clinic at regular intervals:

- Your doctor can check that your control remains as good as it can be.

- If the tests are erratic or show high sugar levels, your doctor will be able to explain the changes you need to make.

- He will wish to be sure that your tests remain a reliable indicator of good control. It is now possible to perform tests which can assess your average control.

- Your doctor will have the opportunity to check on your ability to cope with day-to-day problems.

- They provide you with an opportunity to ask questions and discuss any new problems.

- Finally, and most importantly, every so often, particularly after you have had diabetes for ten years or so, your eyes, feet and kidney function will be tested, in case you need treatment for any of the late complications of diabetes. As these late complications can and should be detected by your doctor well before you notice any problems, visits to the clinic are <u>essential.</u>

Diabetes and other illnesses

The effect of illness on diabetes

In the section on treatment (Chapter 3) it was indicated that under certain circumstances your diabetes may go temporarily out of control. Although a few days' loss of control is of no real significance, if you should develop symptoms of <u>thirst</u> and <u>dryness of the mouth</u>, or <u>pass large quantities of urine</u>, you should consult your doctor.

Diabetes and the treatment of other illnesses

Diabetes is no bar to the treatment — including operations — of any other disorder or illness. Because your diabetes may not be so easily controlled during a period of sickness, your doctor may be selective in prescribing treatment.

Dentistry

Straightforward, routine dental treatment can be carried out by your dentist in the normal way. When the treatment involves general anaesthesia, however, then this should always be performed by a hospital team and not in the dental surgery.

For all routine dental procedures, **INSULIN MUST BE ADMINISTERED AS USUAL** — it must not be stopped or reduced for fear that insufficient food will be taken to balance it. The reason for this is that the stress of the procedure is likely to raise the blood sugar, rather than lower it.

```
TELEPHONE                              22B HIGH STREET
BRIGHTON 7401                          BRIGHTON
                                       SUSSEX

                    Dental Surgeon
        Ernest D W Day (B.D.S., L.D.S., R.C.S.)
                Your next appointment is:

            January 7th  4.30 p.m.
            June 22nd  3.00 p.m.
```

If you are unable to take the normal portions of food, then these should be replaced with fluids containing sugar in equivalent amounts, until you are eating normally again. Should you have any doubts about a planned dental procedure, discuss it with your doctor before going ahead.

Diabetic control whilst in hospital

When you are in hospital you are usually confined to bed and will not be taking any exercise. Also you will be anxious, and your diet will most probably be different. Together, these factors will undoubtedly cause your blood sugar to rise and your tests to become positive. Consequently, your insulin dose will need to be increased. You should realize that the cause of these changes in your diabetic control is the result of prevailing circumstances, and not a failure on your part or on the part of the hospital staff.

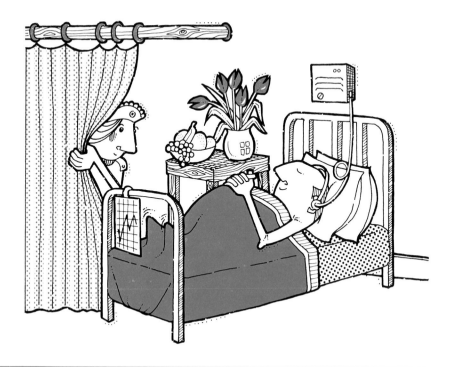

Diabetes and the partially sighted

If you have difficulty in seeing or are blind, you may have problems with the various techniques required to control your diabetes, i.e. insulin injections, urine tests and blood tests.

Injections

There are various devices available to help you with your injections. For those with mild to moderate impairment there is a magnifying glass which can fit onto the syringe to enlarge the markings.

For those with more severe loss of vision two devices are available:

- A pre-set syringe, suitable for those in whom the dose is seldom varied
- A click count syringe, suitable for those mixing insulins and varying their doses. This consists of a syringe with a ratchet in which the units of insulin drawn into the syringe can be counted by listening to or feeling the clicks which are produced as the plunger is drawn back. There is also a device for helping to locate the needle of the syringe into the neck of the insulin bottle.

Urine and blood testing

Standard urine and blood tests depend on visual comparisons and clearly cannot be performed by people with marked visual impairment (or those with certain types of colour blindness). To help with this a meter has been marketed by Hypoguard for urine and blood testing, which enables the test strips to be located by feel and which indicates the values by audible signals. With the aid of these devices, many partially sighted people with diabetes find it possible to give their own injections and monitor themselves. In cases of severe difficulty, however, support should be sought from the district nurse, social services and health visitors.

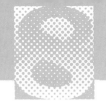

MARRIAGE

Should those with diabetes get married?

Young people with diabetes often ask whether it is wise to get married. The answer is almost always 'Yes'.

It is only fair that the non-diabetic partner should want to know something about diabetes, and be reassured about the likely effects it could have on the marriage.

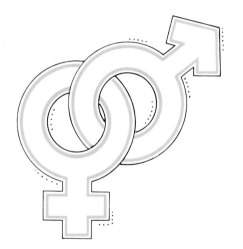

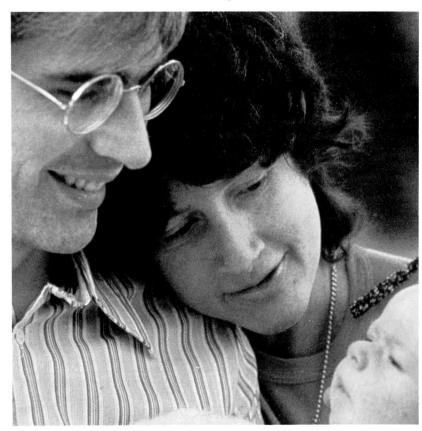

Fig. 8.1
Diabetes should not prevent you from getting married and having a family.

Sexual development

You may often worry about the possibility that your diabetes may prevent you from having a normal sexual life. However, worry is far more likely to upset your sex life than the diabetes! If your diabetes is well controlled, you should have no more problems than anybody else.

Puberty will occur normally — almost everybody feels that they have not developed as well as others of the same age, whether they have diabetes or not! Very occasionally, if somebody has only just developed diabetes, or has had a series of high sugar tests, puberty may be delayed slightly. Should this happen in your case, do not worry, everything will work properly eventually.

Remember that sexual intercourse is a form of exercise too — it is a well-known and sometimes embarrassing cause of hypoglycaemia.

Is someone with diabetes normally fertile?

The answer is 'Yes', although, of course, there are exceptions. In the days before insulin was discovered, few women with diabetes conceived, and even fewer had live babies. It may still be true that a woman whose diabetes is very badly controlled might have some difficulty in conceiving, but where the condition is reasonably well controlled, conception should be normal.

Nor is there any reason why a healthy man with diabetes should not be able to father children. As with women, very badly controlled diabetes can temporarily lessen a man's fertility. Occasionally, diabetes can lead to impotence, but this usually happens very much later in life.

Should a woman with diabetes have children?

If a woman is going to have a baby, she should be able to care for the child until it is grown up and able to lead an independent life. Should she have any serious complications — particularly complications involving the kidneys — the couple ought to think very carefully before embarking on a pregnancy. If there are no complications, or only minor ones, then there should be no bar to pregnancy on account of the diabetes.

"Will our child get diabetes?"

This is perhaps the commonest question asked. The simple answer is 'No', because the likelihood of a baby being born with permanent diabetes is zero.

"But will my child develop diabetes, say at the age of 5 or 10?" Again, the answer is encouraging. The chances of your child developing diabetes in childhood, although greater than normal, (but still only something like 1 in 100 as opposed to the normal 1 in 500), are still unlikely. By this reckoning, 99 out of every 100 children will not develop diabetes, and it would appear that most couples would consider this to be an acceptable risk.

You must remember that the answers to these questions are not certainties, they are only probabilities; one can never be sure that anyone will or will not get diabetes.

Diabetes and menstruation

Diabetes can have an effect on menstruation, particularly if the diabetes is poorly controlled. In such cases, periods may be upset, scanty, or missed altogether. But the most likely cause of a missed period is pregnancy!

Menstruation can have an effect on your diabetes. For instance, periods sometimes cause a variation in the blood sugar, and you may notice a definite change in the results of your blood or urine tests for a few days. If these changes are regular, there is no harm in increasing or decreasing your insulin dosage for a day or two, as indicated by the blood tests.

PREGNANCY

A woman with diabetes needs special care during her pregnancy, and she should make every endeavour to keep her diabetes fully under control. In the past, about a third of the babies born to women with diabetes were lost. Now, with good care, the chances of losing a baby are only very slightly greater than for those women who do not have diabetes.

Before becoming pregnant

If you intend to start a family, or have another child, you should inform your GP, or the doctor at your diabetic clinic, just in case there should be any medical reason why you should not become pregnant. You should then try to get the best possible control of your diabetes — usually this necessitates two injections daily, possibly with a mixture of insulins — so that the newly conceived baby will start its development under the best possible conditions. The reason for this special emphasis on good control before pregnancy is that babies are occasionally born with abnormalities, and this is slightly more common in babies born to those with diabetes. If the diabetic control is near-perfect, then the chance of any of these abnormalities occurring is very small. If the father has diabetes, his control does not increase this risk.

Control of diabetes during pregnancy

Keeping perfect control

Once pregnancy is confirmed, you should aim to achieve and maintain very good control. Fortunately, this becomes easier as the pregnancy proceeds. The aim is to achieve blood sugar levels between 4 and 8 mmol/l, even after meals. It is usually best for a pregnant woman to be cared for at a hospital with a special diabetic clinic. During your pregnancy, it will probably be necessary for you to visit the clinic every 2 to 4 weeks, in order that your diabetic control can be carefully monitored.

Monitoring your control

Frequent tests are important and must be performed carefully during pregnancy. Your urine tests may become positive, because sugar often leaks into the urine rather more easily than usual (the blood sugar remaining normal). Therefore, during pregnancy, urine tests may be unreliable, and if your tests become positive, you should always have a blood test before increasing your insulin dose. In fact, regular blood testing avoids this problem and is normally recommended. Poor control could necessitate your being admitted to hospital for a few days, in order to ensure a rapid return to good control.

When you and your doctor are trying to get very tight control of your diabetes, there may be a slightly greater risk of hypoglycaemia than usual. This will cause your baby no harm.

Insulin dosage during pregnancy

Your insulin requirement is likely to increase during pregnancy, especially in the second half, when the demand could increase by 50-100% or even more. However, you need not conclude that your diabetes is worse. The dose of insulin always falls to the pre-pregnancy amount immediately after the baby is born.

Diabetes developing during pregnancy

Occasionally, diabetes is discovered for the first time during pregnancy, as a result of the routine tests which all pregnant women undergo. The treatment of this 'gestational diabetes' as it is called, is exactly the same as for long-standing diabetes. In the majority of such cases the problem is almost always resolved as soon as the baby has been delivered, and no further treatment is required. However, this type of diabetes will recur with subsequent pregnancies, and any woman who has had this problem with her first child should always report to her doctor at once, if she thinks she is pregnant again.

Hospital admission

Most hospitals recommend that women with diabetes are admitted a week or so before their baby is due, so that a very careful check can be made on diabetic control and on the baby's progress. Delivery is often earlier than the expected time of birth, because some babies born to women with diabetes tend to be heavier than normal, and if they go the full forty weeks, their size may make labour difficult. However, if tests of the baby's development show that it is not large, then the pregnancy may be allowed to go the full term before delivery. These tests involve the technique of ultrasound, by means of which it is possible to measure the baby's size accurately.

Sometimes, a sample of amniotic fluid (the fluid around the baby in the womb) will be taken, in order to make sure that the baby is developing normally.

The method of delivery

The method of delivery will be influenced by many factors. Normal, vaginal delivery is preferable, but if a woman has previously had a Caesarian section, or if the baby is large or shows any signs of distress during labour, then a Caesarian section is usually performed.

Controlling your diabetes during labour

During labour an intravenous drip (a tube is inserted in a vein in the arm) is nearly always set up. Via this tube your diabetes will be carefully controlled in one of two ways:

- A continuous insulin infusion, either with a special pump, or by adding insulin to the saline (salt water) which is being given through the drip
- Provision of sugar water in case you are not eating normally.

Blood sugar measurements will be carried out every hour or two, in order to check that your diabetes is being adequately controlled. Very soon after your baby has been born, the drip will be stopped, and insulin will be given by injection twice a day.

The first few days

For the first few hours or days after the birth, your baby may need intensive care in a special neonatal ward. This will be necessary if, for example:

- The birth has been difficult
- Your baby is large

In most cases, however, babies born to parents with diabetes are healthy from the start, and there should be no reason why your baby should not be with you and be cared for in the same way as other new-born babies.

The first few weeks

Your baby may be born a little heavier than average, and his or her weight gain may be less in the first few weeks than expected. Indeed, some weight loss may occur, but don't be alarmed if this happens.

- If you plan to become pregnant, try to balance your diabetes as well as possible.
- Consult your doctor or clinic, preferably before you conceive and certainly as soon as you become pregnant.
- Test regularly and carefully.
- Adjust your insulin to achieve blood test results of 4 to 8 mmol/l.

Controlling your diabetes when you get home from hospital will require a little more effort than it did before your baby was born.

Immediately your baby has been delivered, your insulin requirements will fall. Therefore, the day following the birth you should return to the type and dose of insulin you were taking before you became pregnant. If you only started taking insulin during the pregnancy, the chances are that once your baby is born you can stop having injections altogether.

What about breast feeding?

There is no reason why you should not breast feed your baby, if you so choose. However, if you do breast feed, you will need to take extra carbohydrate to compensate for loss of sugar in the breast milk. In addition, night feeds will mean that you are working harder. You must have your snacks regularly, and you may need extra carbohydrate at night. Feed your baby and yourself at the same time.

Should blood tests be continued?

If you were taught how to perform blood tests during pregnancy, you should continue with them, although the number of tests can be reduced. It is essential for your continued good health that you try to maintain the very good control established during pregnancy, and blood tests can prove invaluable in this respect.

How many children should a woman with diabetes have?

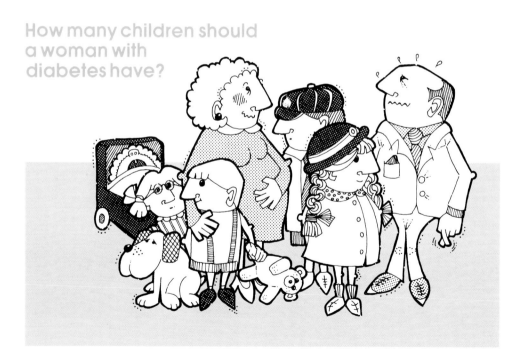

There is no definite answer to this question. The need for extra care during pregnancy, and the need for admission to hospital towards the end of pregnancy, may be good reasons for restricting the size of the family. Furthermore, after two Caesarian sections, most obstetricians would advise against any more pregnancies. In the end, of course, the decision must rest with the parents.

Adoption

There is no particular reason why someone with insulin dependent diabetes, and who has no late complications, should not adopt a child. Adoption agencies do, however, require that prospective parents are fit and well, and that they have a responsible attitude to their diabetes.

CONTRACEPTION

Which type of contraceptive?

There are no forms of contraception which are forbidden, or known to be particularly harmful, to diabetic women. Nonetheless, some forms do seem to be slightly better than others.

The cap and sheath

Using these forms of contraception poses no problems.

Intrauterine devices

The 'coil' seems to be a satisfactory form of contraception for those with diabetes, though slightly less safe than the cap or sheath. In many women the coil has remained in position for a year or more, but there does appear to be a slightly greater risk of inflammation or infection in those with diabetes.

The 'pill'

The 'pill' is the most convenient form of contraception, but is not suitable for everyone. Those with a raised blood pressure, or thrombosis, should not take the pill.

Generally speaking, there is little or no risk involved in a young woman taking the pill for short periods — say, a year or so. For longer term use, however, there is a slightly increased risk of accelerating blood vessel complications. For this reason it may be preferable to use the 'mini' or progesterone-only pill, the use of which appears not to carry such risks.

If you take the usual type of pill, which contains oestrogen, you may find that your blood sugar rises a little, so that you may need to adjust your insulin dose.

Sterilization

Sterilization in women, by tying the Fallopian tubes, or in men, by vasectomy, can be performed as easily and as safely in those with diabetes as in those without diabetes.

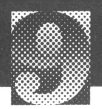
One of the main aims of your treatment is that it should interfere as little as possible with your day-to-day activities. Nonetheless, some modifications will undoubtedly be necessary.

Employment

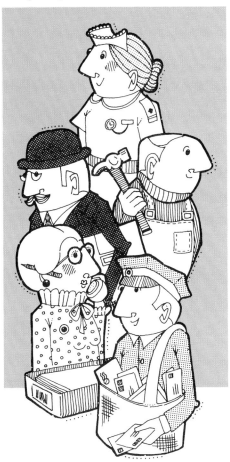

Jobs which can be done by those on insulin

The vast majority of people taking insulin are able to continue, or take up, work in the normal way. There should be no impairment of your ability to function as well as — if not better than — you did before you developed diabetes.

Almost all types of occupation are open to people taking insulin, with the exception of jobs where development of hypoglycaemia could put other people at risk. These jobs are described below:

● You are not allowed to fly aeroplanes, or hold a Public Service Vehicle licence nor usually a Heavy Goods Vehicle licence. These restrictions have been imposed to safeguard other people, since if you were to have a reaction your vehicle could go out of control.

● The Armed Services, the Police Force, and the Fire Service require strict standards of health. Whereas you might be perfectly all right if you have a hypoglycaemic reaction, other peoples' safety could be seriously jeopardized. Consequently, these Services do not accept those with insulin dependent diabetes. If, however, you develop diabetes while in service, you will not necessarily need to retire, but may be able to transfer to less hazardous duties.

● If you have a potentially dangerous job, such as deep-sea diving, or steeplejacking, you will probably have to change your job. If you never have reactions you may think such a step is unnecessary. However, simply ask yourself — "If I should have a reaction when doing my job, could I harm myself or cause injury to other people"? If the answer is "Yes", then perhaps you should consider an alternative career.

Applying for a job

It is often felt that employers may discriminate against people with diabetes. When this occurs, it is usually as a result of the employer being misinformed or unaware of the true facts about diabetes. Usually, however, if you are the best applicant, you will very likely get the job. If you should find that your explanations are not being accepted, then you should consider asking your doctor to talk to your would-be employer. Alternatively, you could ask your doctor to provide a reference prior to making your job application. When an employer appreciates the self-discipline you require in order to control your diabetes, then he may consider you to be a rather better bet than some of the other applicants. This is confirmed by the above average work record of most people with diabetes. You may be tempted to conceal the fact that you have diabetes — don't, it may only cause problems later, especially if you have an unexpected hypoglycaemic reaction.

How diabetes affects your job

To carry out your job effectively you will need to keep your diabetes well controlled. It will be necessary for you to have regular breaks for snacks, and to have your meals on time. This should be explained to your employer, together with the fact that you could suffer a hypoglycaemic reaction. You should, however, reassure your employer, by stressing that:

- Most hypoglycaemic attacks are prevented by eating regularly. Usually, they are very short-lived, and are easily relieved within a minute or so, by taking sugar or its equivalent.

- Severe attacks involving loss of consciousness are extremely rare.

- The dangers to which you might be exposed when working with machinery are minimal, and the warning symptoms of hypoglycaemia will prevent major incidents.

Driving a car or van (but not a Public Services Vehicle or a Heavy Goods Vehicle) should be no problem, providing that you do not have severe hypoglycaemic reactions without warning (see Driving, page 134).

It is also extremely important that your work colleagues know that you have diabetes. If, for example, they detect symptoms of hypoglycaemia before you do, then they can alert you; it will also prove very useful if they know exactly what to do if you should have an exceptionally bad attack.

The vast majority of people with diabetes should not regard themselves as disabled. Only very rarely should someone with diabetes be registered as 'Disabled' with the Disablement Resettlement Officer at the local Job Centre. If, however, you have developed any physical disabilities, or have severe frequent and uncontrolled reactions without warning, then this may be necessary.

Starting work for the first time

You may have discovered that you needed less insulin when at school than when you were on holiday. Likewise, you will find that when working, especially if your job involves manual labour, you will probably need to reduce your insulin. It is a wise precaution, therefore, to reduce your insulin slightly on the day you start work. Take some tests and if the sugar level is low, have an extra portion of carbohydrates.

It is essential that you continue to take your snacks at the correct time. You may feel embarrassed to ask for breaks when your colleagues continue working, but it is much more embarrassing to have a hypoglycaemic reaction. Always choose food which is small, and easily chewed and swallowed.

When you start work you may find that your injection and breakfast times will have to be earlier than when you were at school. If that is the case, you should bring forward the time of your snack. If your work routine is very different from your school routine — very early or very late shifts, for instance — some changes may need to be made to your insulin dosage and type.

Financial considerations

Insurance

On all insurance proposals where data are required for underwriting assessment, it is imperative that statements are made in good faith, and that there is a full disclosure of material facts. If it transpires that there has been non-disclosure of <u>any</u> material fact, then the contract can be repudiated. On most proposals, specific questions are asked to elicit certain information, and for many types of insurance, diabetes is a fact which underwriters will wish to consider. Disclosure will enable the insurer to ask for supplementary information, to seek a report from your doctor, or to ask for a medical examination if it is considered necessary.

In assessing a risk, different insurers take different views. The British Diabetic Association's brokers will be particularly helpful, because they will not only be able to advise you on the type of cover best suited to your specific needs, but also, by virtue of many years of experience in dealing with insurance problems, they will be able to select the insurers with the most realistic underwriting views according to the type of cover required.

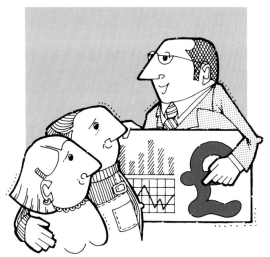

Life assurance

Because of the possibility of long-term complications, it is usual for some premium loading to be placed on life assurance. The loading applied to term assurance, such as mortgage protection, is likely to be higher than that applied to whole life or endowment policies.

Motor insurance

You are advised in the section on Driving, page 134, about the need for full and honest statements to insurance companies.

Your insurer may ask for an additional premium, although many companies will quote normal rates, providing you have not been involved in an accident attributable to your diabetes.

Permanent sickness and accident insurance

When people with diabetes seek this type of insurance they are likely to have to pay higher than normal premiums. A policy suited to people with diabetes is available through the British Diabetic Association's brokers.

Travel and personal accident insurance

This is a field of insurance in which you need to be especially careful. If you take out such a policy, you should pay particular attention to the exclusion clauses, which normally exclude all pre-existing illness. The Association's brokers, however, offer a full cover which does not exclude diabetes. This cover is not available if you are over the age of 75, or in respect of skiing holidays.

Pensions/superannuation

You should not encounter any problems negotiating normal pension and superannuation rights.

Other financial considerations

- Prescription charges in the U.K. are waived for all people taking insulin. A form (CP11) will be signed by your doctor, which will enable you to obtain an exemption certificate. This applies to all prescriptions, whether related to your diabetes or not.

- Your diet should not involve you in any additional expense. If your expenditure has increased, however, and this is creating difficulties, discussion with your dietitian and local Social Security Office may enable you to obtain some help.

- Travel to hospital clinics, if frequent, may be a financial problem. Again, help can often by obtained by discussion with your doctor or hospital social worker.

- Those who develop late complications , especially with their eyes, may be eligible for additional benefits.

Fig. 9.1
Keeping fit is an essential aspect of maintaining good control of your diabetes.

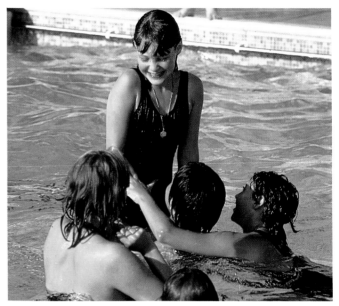

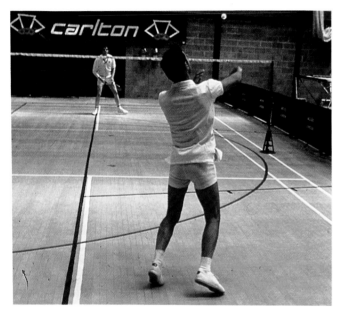

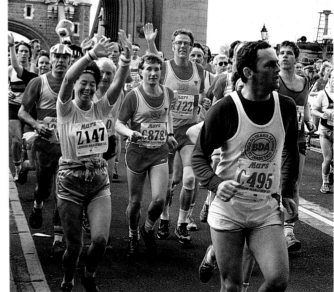

Sport and outdoor activities

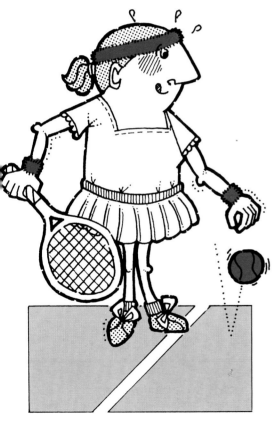

Which sports and activities are prohibited?

There are very few sports in which those on insulin have not competed or even excelled. Athletics of all kinds, first class professional football, mountaineering, marathon running and the usual activities of a less tiring type, such as gardening and walking, are all within the capabilities of people on insulin.

Therefore, it must be stressed that, with one or two exceptions, you should not give up your sporting activities. Indeed, good physical fitness will help your diabetic control by making the action of insulin on your fat and muscle cells more efficient. The only requirement is that you take simple but essential precautions, as already described in Chapter 6, page 92.

Strenuous activity, such as swimming, football or heavy manual work, use up sugar, with the result that unless you have more carbohydrate or reduce your insulin dose you will have a hypo. It is not sensible to alter your insulin every day or so, to suit this sort of activity — and, in any case, you will still need to eat more if you take a lot of exercise. Thus, it is better to increase your carbohydrate intake than to change your insulin dose. The amount of extra carbohydrate needed varies from person to person, and is also influenced by the strenuousness of the activity. You should certainly allow an extra 20 g for swimming, and more if you are a distance swimmer. Four-strip Kit Kats and mini Mars Bars are quickly absorbed, and are quite suitable as an extra snack. For ball games, such as football, make sure you have some extra carbohydrate at half-time, and carry glucose sweets or Dextrosol in your pockets for emergencies. The same principles apply when starting work, especially hard manual work (see page 119). With prolonged exercise you will need to replenish your energies after an hour or so. If the exercise occurs on a regular basis, for example, if you are an athlete in training, or you play sport professionally, a regular reduction in insulin dosage is sensible.

If you take all the necessary precautions, strenuous activities should not cause any serious problems. For example, if you should have a hypo while playing football, no great harm will result. Simply, sit down, have some glucose and play again when you feel better.

Where caution is necessary

There are two types of sport where you need to exercise special care: those which may be termed 'risky' sports, and those where you might drive yourself to exhaustion. 'Risky' sports — swimming, sub-aqua diving, hang gliding, solo sailing or mountaineering — are clearly not advisable if you are prone to hypoglycaemia. You would not be able to eat a lump of sugar while hanging below a glider and therefore might lapse into unconsciousness! As with work, you should always ask yourself: "If I develop hypoglycaemia while doing X, could I take my sugar; if not, would I be in danger and would I put anybody else at risk?"

In all high-risk activities you need to take extra precautions. They may seem obvious enough, but in the excitement of the moment they are easily forgotten, perhaps at considerable cost. Taking rock climbing and mountaineering as examples, here is what you should do:

- Measure your blood glucose before setting off
- Take emergency supplies of insulin and glucose
- Take enough food for twice as long as you think you will be away
- Since there will be other people with you, split the emergency supplies between you, so that if your rucksack drops off the rock face, all is not lost.

Swimming is another potentially risky sport, and you should always follow these simple rules:

- Never go swimming alone
- Whoever accompanies you swimming must know how to treat a hypo and have the means to do so
- Never go swimming at times when hypoglycaemia is most likely to occur — just before a meal, for example
- Have a "swimming snack" before your start.

Thus, the message is simple: whilst reactions are unpleasant and should be prevented if at all possible, they are truly dangerous only if they occur in a potentially dangerous situation, such as when in a swimming bath.

Sports which can lead to exhaustion — marathon running and professional sports — are not prohibited, but special care is necessary if you are to avoid getting very short of fuel or liquid. By supplementing your diet carefully and replenishing your 'fuel stores', you should manage very well, but if you have problems, talk to your doctor.

Travel, holidays and diabetes

You should be able to travel on holiday or business, either in this country or abroad, in exactly the same way as anybody else.

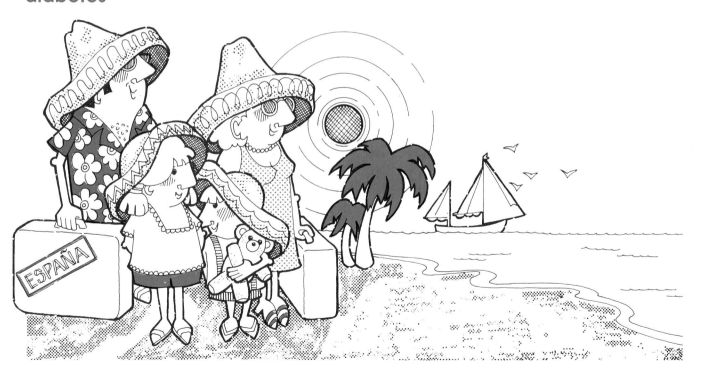

Who should know that you have diabetes?

If you are not travelling with your family, you should make sure that any travelling companions not only know that you have diabetes, but also exactly what to do in an emergency. They should know where you keep your glucose, and be aware of the need to seek medical help in an emergency. It could also be helpful if they know how to give an injection of insulin if, say, you were to injure your arm in a skiing accident, or an injection of glucagon (see Chapter 6 page 91 and Appendix 4, page 201), if you were very hypoglycaemic.

When travelling by air, it is wise to let members of the crew know that you have diabetes.

Identification

In case of language difficulties, always carry your diabetic identity card, and preferably one translated into the language of the country you are visiting.

Vaccinations

You can be vaccinated, and are able to take other preventative measures, in the same way as someone without diabetes.

Travel sickness

You should always remind yourself when planning a journey that even though travel is commonplace, journeys are not always smooth, literally or metaphorically. Travel sickness may be a hazard, and if you are prone to it you should ask your doctor beforehand for tablets. Kwells are mild but safe, whereas antihistamines are stronger but may make you drowsy.

If you are the sort of person who suffers from travel sickness, always take some sweetened fruit juices, which you should drink instead of your normal portions. You should also take the usual steps to increase your insulin if your tests indicate an increase in blood sugar.

Your insulin and syringe

You should always carry your insulin and syringe with you in your hand luggage. This is allowed by airlines, and you should always refuse to give them to anyone, even if they promise to give them to the cabin staff for safe-keeping until you need them.

Always carry a spare syringe and other supplies in your main baggage, in case your hand luggage is lost or stolen.

To avoid any problems, particularly with Customs or police, you should always have some formal means of identifying yourself as having diabetes, such as a B.D.A. card, Medicalert, or S.O.S. bracelets or necklaces.

Syringes

Many prefer to buy disposable syringes for use when away from home on business or holiday. For a long holiday, however, a glass syringe in a spirit-proof case may be much less bulky. Whatever you prefer, ensure that you have enough supplies to last not only the duration of your holiday but longer, in case you should be delayed.

Insulin availability

Insulin is available in all developed countries and in most others as well, at least in the main cities. But, because the type, strength and purity may differ from your usual insulin, it is best to take adequate amounts with you. If, however, you are going to reside abroad for, say, one or two years, you should enquire beforehand as to the availability of supplies locally. Your N.H.S. family doctor is not allowed to give you a bulk supply of insulin if you intend to reside abroad for some months, but he can give you enough to see you through any reasonable holiday period.

In Canada, U.S.A. and Australia the same strengths of insulin are available as in the U.K., but in most other countries different strengths are used.

Insulin will remain fully active for at least one month at a temperature of 25°C (77°F). Thus, it is only in very hot climates that you will have to ensure satisfactory refrigeration (not freezing) for your reserve supplies. However, insulin stored in the glove compartment or on the dash board or rear window ledge of a car left in full sunshine will rapidly deteriorate, not only in Mediterranean countries, but even in Scotland! In tropical countries keep your insulin in a pre-cooled vacuum flask when travelling.

Dehydration

If you visit countries with tropical or very hot climates you will sweat more than when at home, and this may cause a significant loss of salt and water which, if severe, will cause sunstroke (more correctly called heat stroke). This is a hazard for everyone newly arrived in the tropics, but with diabetes could lead to a serious loss of fluid. Therefore, it is important, to take a few simple precautions:

- Maintain an adequate supply of water and salt
- Do not over-exert yourself
- Wear loose-fitting and comfortable clothing
- Keep your body covered and avoid sunburn.

Sickness

One of the commonest problems among travellers is diarrhoea. Very rarely, it may be due to a serious infection, such as typhoid or paratyphoid fever, or even cholera. Vaccination offers some protection against these, but, in addition, it is essential to take adequate hygiene and preventative measures, and these will also be of some help against the less serious, but still troublesome and very much more common, 'traveller's tummy':

- Do not drink unbottled water unless you boil it or add sterilizing tablets
- Avoid uncooked foods and vegetables and fruit you have not peeled
- If you eat shellfish, make sure they are fresh and well cooked
- Avoid all foods which have been cooked and then cooled, such as cold buffets or puddings
- Obtain some antibiotic tablets from your doctor before leaving,

and take these according to his instructions.

In the case of illness, you should follow your usual precautions and increase your insulin, if necessary, but never reduce it. Fortunately, most tummy upsets are of short duration, and are nearly always due to a change in diet, so that with care you should be able to manage without medical help.

Availability of medical assistance

This is rarely free. Countries in the EEC have reciprocal medical cover, but before you go you must fill in a Form E.111, available from your local DSS office, in order to get the necessary certificate to prove you are eligible for the treatment. Even then, the cover may not be as comprehensive as in this country. Thus, it is essential, especially where no reciprocal arrangement exists, to take out adequate medical insurance. If you should experience any difficulty in obtaining this type of insurance, the British Diabetic Association's insurance brokers can help you (address available from the Diabetes Care Department of the B.D.A.).

Finally, always carry a card indicating that you have diabetes requiring insulin treatment (see Fig. 6.2, page 90).

Air travel

Most airlines provide food very frequently — sometimes too often — and since you will not be taking much exercise and will probably be more excited than usual, you could be slightly 'sugary' for a few days. This will do you no harm, and at least you can be fairly confident that you will not become hypoglycaemic.

On long journeys, in particular, it is wise to tell the cabin staff if you have diabetes.

Your insulin and time changes

The only problems you are likely to face are with time zone changes when on long flights. Travelling west prolongs the day, travelling east shortens it, and this can cause problems for those taking insulin. How you cope, depends on the type and dosage of your insulin (Figs 9.2 and 9.3).

Fig. 9.2
What you should do when crossing
time zones if you take a single,
daily injection of long-acting insulin.

SINGLE, LONG-ACTING INSULIN INJECTIONS

If you are on a single, long-acting insulin injection, you may find it easier to keep your watch on British time when setting out (or on the time of the country of departure when returning). Eat your regular meals according to this time until you arrive, when you should adjust to suit the local time.

Going eastwards

You will find that the day is shortened, so that your next injection will appear to be due less than 24 hours after the last one.

What should you do?

Take extra carbohydrate with the meal after your next injection, in case there is insulin left over from the previous one.

Going westwards

The day will become longer. You will probably have an extra meal in the day.

What should you do?

Give yourself a little extra insulin initially, and eat meals every 3 hours to prevent hypoglycaemia. In case this should happen, always carry some sugar with you — and too much rather than too little.
OR
Make no changes. If on the second day you are more 'sugary', increase your next insulin injection a little.

Fig. 9.3
What you should do when crossing
time zones if you inject insulin twice
daily.

TWICE-DAILY INSULIN INJECTIONS

Going eastwards

The day is shorter.

What should you do?

Give your normal morning injection and reduce the evening injection by 10%. For flights of more than 24 hours you may find it easier to give yourself more frequent, smaller — say half the usual — doses of quick-acting (clear) insulin before each meal.

Going westwards

The day is longer.

What should you do?

After your second 'evening' injection, which will be needed at 6-7pm British time, you may still be up and eating five or six hours later. Therefore, take another small — say half your usual — dose of clear insulin six hours after the second injection and follow this with a meal.

Testing

If you usually use Clinitest tablets it would be worth changing to Diastix or Diabur for the journey, since they do not require any test tubes or the addition of water.

Blood glucose monitoring is, of course, feasible, either with your usual 'stick' or with a meter. If you are away for several weeks, a voltage adapter may be necessary to recharge your meter.

Finally, don't let your diabetes put you off travelling.

Emigration

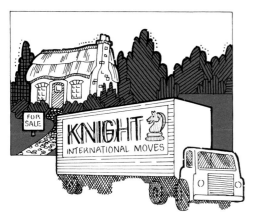

Uncomplicated diabetes should be no bar to emigration. A certificate of health is normally required, and you will need a statement from your doctor to say that your diabetes is reasonably well controlled. There may be more problems if you suffer from any of the complications of diabetes, such as visual impairment or foot problems, but this will need to be discussed with the emigration department concerned or your own doctor. In either case, remember that health care in the country you are going to may not be free, and you should, therefore, take out the appropriate health insurance cover. You should also take a letter from your doctor, containing details of your treatment. Remember, too, that some countries may not be using U100 insulin, in which case you will require a change of insulin strength and syringe.

Social life

Evening parties, discos and dances

Delaying the evening injection is a frequent occurrence if you are to enjoy an active social life. So, what do you do if you are invited to a party, at which the meal is planned for, say, 8pm, when you normally have your evening injection at 5.30pm and your meal at 6.00pm?

The answer is straightforward:

- Delay your injection until 7.30pm.
- Have a 10 g snack at your normal evening meal time (fruit juice is quick-acting and will not spoil your appetite).
- Assume the meal will be late and be prepared to have an extra snack if the meal is very late.

If you have only one injection a day, 'reverse' the evening meal and bed-time snack, so that you have a 20g snack, say at 6pm, to tide you over until the meal at 8pm.

When you go to a party or disco:

- Try to have your evening injection and meal at the usual time.

- If the party or disco starts early, and food and drink are available, you can save 2 or 3 portions of your carbohydrate allowance from the evening meal to have during the party. Add these portions to your usual allowance for evening or bed-time snacks.
- Add a further 4 or 5 portions if you dance like a maniac; 2 or 3 portions for a lively performance; and nothing if you just sit and watch!

Don't let your diabetes put you off dancing — enjoy yourself!

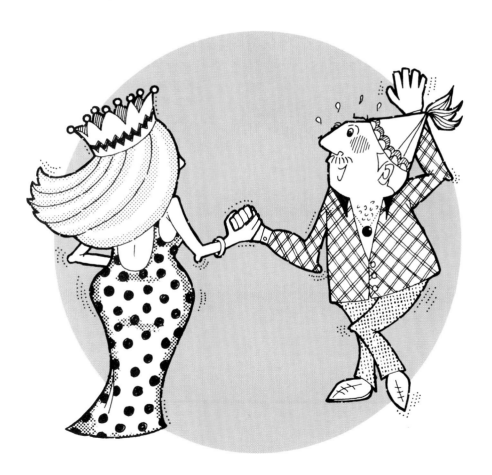

Driving

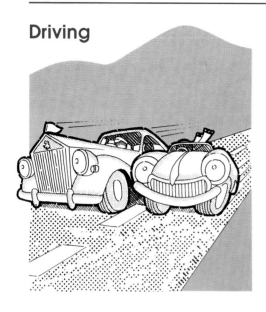

Points to remember

You must:

- Tell your insurance company that you have diabetes.
- Tell the licensing authorities (D.V.L.C., Swansea, SA99 1AT) that you have diabetes.

Filling in the licence application form

When you apply for a driving licence you have to answer one question of particular importance to you — Question 6(e) asks:

> "Have you now or have you ever had: epilepsy or sudden attacks of disabling giddiness or fainting or any mental illness or defect or any other disability which could affect your fitness as a driver either now or in the future?"

To this question you should answer 'Yes', whether you have diabetes treated with insulin, tablets or diet alone. In the space provided for details, you should state that you have diabetes, adding that your diabetes is controlled by diet/tablets/insulin as appropriate. After you have completed and returned your application form, you may be sent a supplementary form, asking for further information, including the name and address of your doctor or hospital clinic, as well as your consent for the Driver and Vehicle Licensing Centre to approach your doctor direct. This complication of procedure does not mean that you will be refused a driving licence. The licence will normally be issued for three years and renewals will be made free of charge.

If your diabetes has been diagnosed only recently and you hold a 'life' licence, this will be revoked and replaced with a 'period' licence. Renewals can take several weeks, but should your licence pass its expiry date you can continue to drive, providing you have made application for a renewal.

Insurance cover

It is compulsory by law for every driver to be insured against the risk of liability for injury to third parties. Most insurers are willing to offer insurance cover to those with diabetes, but some may wish to charge a higher premium. Some insurers will require a medical report from your doctor, who is entitled to charge a fee for this service. If you have difficulty with insurance, the British Diabetic Association can help and advise you.

You must tell your insurers that you have diabetes, no matter how questions in the insurance proposal form may be phrased. Upon diagnosis, existing policy holders must immediately advise their insurers. If you withhold this information and are then involved in an accident, the insurers could be entitled to repudiate your claim, by making the policy null and void on the grounds of non-disclosure.

When not to drive

You should not drive if:

- You are being started on insulin: you should wait until stabilization is complete
- You have difficulty in recognizing early symptoms of hypoglycaemia
- You have any problems with your eyesight that cannot be corrected by glasses.

Driving heavy goods vehicles and public service vehicles

If you inject insulin you are not allowed to hold Public Service Vehicle (PSV) licences, and are not allowed to hold a Heavy Goods Vehicle (HGV) licence.

Alcohol

Never drink and drive. If you are on insulin, a hypoglycaemic reaction may look like drunkenness; if your breath smells of alcohol, suspicions will be heightened. Furthermore, it should be borne in mind that heavy drinking, particularly of spirits, may provoke hypoglycaemia.

'Diabetic' beers should be used only with great caution if you are a car driver; whilst their carbohydrate value is lower than ordinary beer, their alcohol content can be twice as high, and as little as one pint of a diabetic beer can bring your blood alcohol level above the legal limit.

Hypoglycaemia and driving

The dangers of hypoglycaemia while driving are obvious and you must make sure it never happens. Therefore, never drive for more than two hours without a break for a snack.

As soon as you experience any warning signs:

● Stop the car

● Turn off the ignition

● Leave the driving seat until fully recovered

● Have something to eat. Always keep a supply of biscuits and glucose in the car.

If you are found to be hypoglycaemic when in charge of a motor vehicle, especially if you are involved in an accident, you lose your licence for a minimum of six months. This is a very good reason for keeping your diabetes well controlled. Many people find blood testing invaluable as a means of checking that they are safe to drive, without always taking excess carbohydrate 'just in case'.

There can never be any excuse for a reaction while driving: it can never be due to bad luck, only to bad management.

Diabetes and smoking

The dangers of smoking are well known.

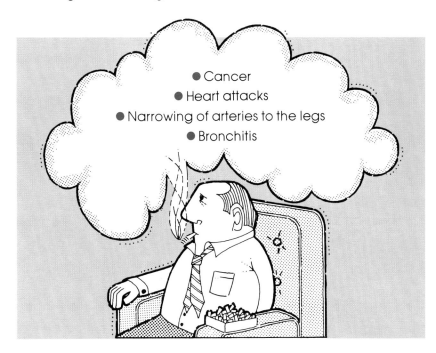

- Cancer
- Heart attacks
- Narrowing of arteries to the legs
- Bronchitis

If you want to avoid these risks, **DON'T SMOKE.**

Diabetes and drugs

It is illegal to possess 'drugs' , such as marijuana, pot, speed, etc. Even so, you may know people who have smoked pot or taken pep pills without coming to any apparent harm. However, for you to take drugs which alter the way your brain works would be dangerous and could possibly be fatal. One of the most serious effects of such drugs is that they cause you to lose your awareness of the warning signs of hypoglycaemia, and at a party where drugs are available it is unlikely that anyone would notice (or care) if you became severely hypoglycaemic. Amphetamine (pep pills) and similar drugs also have a direct effect on diabetes, as well as reducing your awareness of a reaction. So, do not take unnecessary risks by taking drugs which have not been prescribed for you.

Diabetes in children, and parenthood

These topics pose specific problems which, because they are so important, have been covered in their own chapters:

Chapter 8 Marriage, pregnancy, parenthood and contraception.

Chapter 10 Diabetes in children

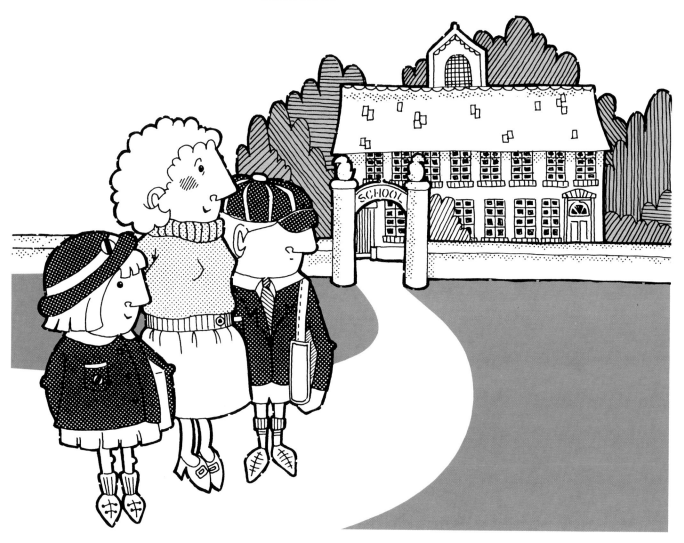

Who is available to help?

From time to time, you may develop problems about which you need specialized advice. On such occasions you may refer to a variety of individuals, including your doctor, nurses, dietitians, chiropodists, the social services and, of course, your local diabetic clinic.

In spite of the help available to you from these specialist individuals and services, you may have additional questions and problems relating to your day-to-day activities, such as careers, insurance, dietary problems etc. This is where the **British Diabetic Association** can be of great assistance.

The BDA has been working to help diabetics for over 50 years. It provides information and advice on all aspects of diabetes. The BDA also acts as spokesman on your behalf, campaigning for better services and to overcome public ignorance and prejudice. Another function of the

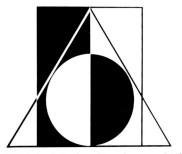

The British Diabetic Association

Association is to support research to help treat, prevent or cure diabetes and its problems.

The BDA has about 350 branches and groups throughout the UK. They hold regular meetings and social events and can give you support locally. Through your local branch you will be able to meet other people with diabetes which may help you to come to terms with everyday problems of living with diabetes.

The Association depends entirely upon voluntary subscriptions and donations, and needs your support. The more members we have, the greater our influence on your behalf.

Fig. 9.4
How the B.D.A. helps and supports those with diabetes.

Nation-wide organization
In the U.K., there are over 350 local groups, which hold regular meetings — everyone is welcome to attend.

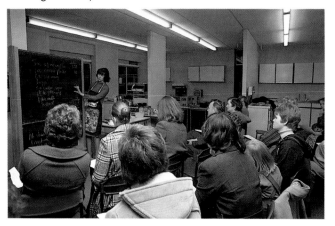

When you have problems
The B.D.A. will provide guidance and help on all problems affecting those with diabetes — but not individual treatment.

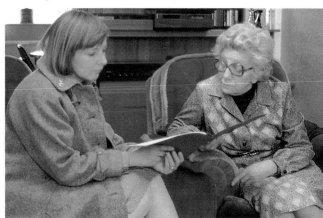

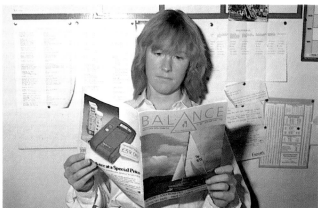

'Balance' a bi-monthly magazine
Members receive 'Balance', the magazine of the B.D.A., free of charge, every two months. It reports progress in medical care and the latest news on legislation that affects those with diabetes. There is information on diets and recipes, articles on personalities and practical hints on day-to-day problems.

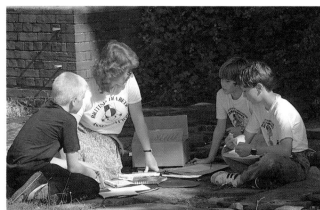

Holidays and advice for young people with diabetes
The Youth Department runs educational and activity holidays for children and teenagers with diabetes. This gives them the opportunity to learn to cope with their problems whilst taking part in normal activities, without being the 'odd one out'. In addition, family teach-in weekends, parents' meetings and international exchanges are all organized. Pen pals are put in touch with each other. Advice is given on careers and other problems. Photo: Chris Schwarz.

Liaison with Government Departments

The Association maintains close contact with Government Departments and other voluntary organizations, to ensure a mutual exchange of information.

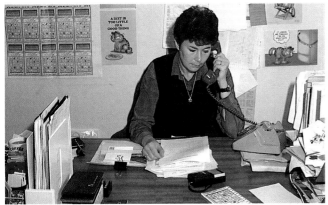

Holidays for adults with diabetes

Summer holidays are organized for adults with diabetes.

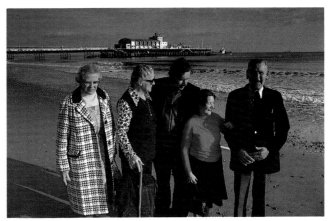

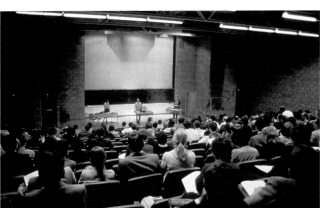

Conferences on diabetes

Through the B.D.A.'s Medical and Scientific, Education and Professional Services Sections, conferences are organized for all people concerned with diabetes, to ensure that they are kept abreast of advances in care and treatment. The B.D.A. is continually striving to make the life of people with diabetes easier and better in every way.

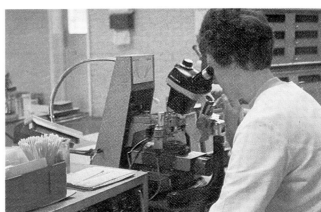

Research

One of the most important aspects of the B.D.A.'s work, certainly the most expensive, is research. The Association is the largest single contributor to diabetic research in the U.K., and currently supports over 60 grants, totalling about £2m.

A final comment

The late Dr. R.D. Lawrence, physician and co-founder of the British Diabetic Association, wrote in his famous book "The Diabetic Life":

> "There is no reason why a diabetic should not, if he can be taught to do so, lead a long and normal life. True, the diabetic life demands self-control from all its subjects, but it gives in return a full and active existence, with no real privations".

The British Diabetic Association
10 Queen Anne Street
London W1M 0BD
Phone: 01-323 1531
Registered Charity No. 215199

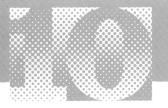

You probably noticed how, after only a few injections, your son or daughter began to look and feel better. In most families, the feeling of relief that all is well is quickly followed by shock or even disbelief that treatment must continue for life, and that for the next few years at least, the treatment will be your direct responsibility.

It is important to stress at the outset, that your child will be able to do all of those things that other children do, and that his or her growth and development should be normal.

Details of insulin dependent diabetes and its treatment have been fully described in the previous chapters, and the information presented there applies equally to children. The same balance should be aimed for, and the adjustments to diet, exercise and insulin are all similar. Therefore, this chapter has been written to provide information on many of the topics which apply specifically to children.

Fig. 10.1
Parents quickly learn the technique of injecting insulin.

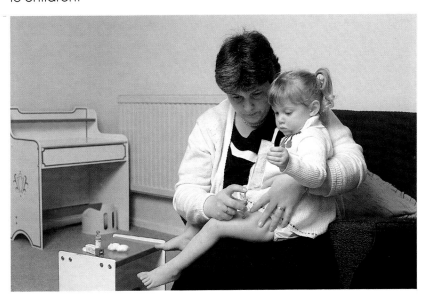

DIABETES AND SMALL CHILDREN

Problems faced by parents

One of the most heart-breaking prospects for parents is the thought of having to give injections. However, having given your child his or her first injection you will have realised that it is not as frightening as you first imagined. But what about your child?

For infants and very young children, it is difficult to explain why injections are necessary. All parents find their own way of coping, and you will be no exception. If there is a secret to success, it is that you should adopt a completely consistent approach to your child, with no attempt at deception or encouragement with false promises that there will be only a few more injections. You will quickly learn that patience, persistence and understanding are the most essential qualities required by the parents of a child with diabetes.

At what age should children inject themselves?

There is no set age by which children must be able to inject themselves, but the sooner the better and, ideally, this should not be later than the move from primary to secondary school.

Therefore, if your child shows the slightest inclination towards carrying out all or part of the injection procedure, without your assistance, then he or she should be encouraged and rewarded for doing so. Many children over the age of 5 or 6 years can give their own injections quite easily (Fig. 10.2) although the parents may wish to check the insulin dose and that it is correctly drawn up. Most children consider that injecting themselves is less painful than being injected by their parents. Having performed their first injection, most children feel proud of their achievement and very often they choose to continue giving their own injections.

As your child grows up and starts to become more independent, there may be a need to spend weekends away at camp or on

Fig. 10.2
Most children over the age of about 6 years are capable of giving their own injections.

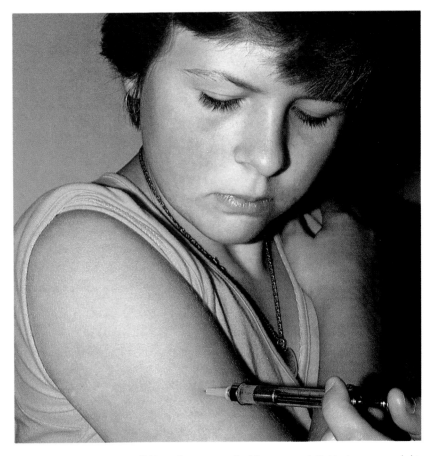

holiday. Clearly, it will then be essential for your child to be capable of performing an injection, and, of course, you will want to feel confident that they will be carried out correctly.

Injection sites and technique

It is as important to inject insulin correctly, as it is to measure the dose accurately. Most children old enough to give their own injections, quickly learn the technique of injecting themselves and do it well for the first few months. Then they discover that injections are less painful if they always inject in the same place. Unfortunately, repeated injections at the same site will eventually damage the skin and underlying tissues, possibly causing an unsightly lump. But worse than the appearance of the injection site is the fact that insulin injected into the lump is not absorbed properly, with the result that control may become sufficiently poor to persuade the unsuspecting parents to increase the dose of insulin. If, on a later occasion, the child tries a new injection site, the larger dose of insulin will be absorbed properly and may cause a hypoglycaemic reaction.

Injections can be given in the thighs, upper arms, buttocks and abdominal wall, but as absorption varies from one site to another, it is suggested that one site should be used for the morning injection and another site used for the evening injection, and that injections should be switched from one side to the other on alternate days (see Appendix 1, Fig. A1.3, page 181).

Injector guns and other aids

Many injection devices (Palmer guns, Hypoguard, Medijet), have been tried, but none has proved entirely satisfactory. British Diabetic Association experience at summer camps for children with diabetes shows that 95 per cent of children do not use injector guns or other aids, and those that do, avoid using them again once they have been taught to inject themselves correctly with a standard syringe. When compared with standard syringes, especially the disposable ones with very fine needles, these pieces of equipment are cumbersome and more difficult to handle. They may, however, help some children to get started, but they are expensive, and parents are advised to seek advice before buying aids of this kind.

Problems of hypoglycaemia in small children

What are the effects of hypoglycaemia in children?

One of the major fears of most parents with a small child with diabetes is that hypoglycaemia might go unrecognized, and that the child could lapse into a deep coma, with perhaps the occurrence of serious brain damage. If you have a very young child, your concern could be even greater, since you probably think that your child will not recognise the symptoms, or will fail to tell you about them. These fears are, however, unwarranted, because the symptoms of hypoglycaemia are usually quite obvious, and if they should occur at night the child almost invariably wakes up. Death or brain damage from hypoglycaemia are unheard of in children. The reason for this is that, although the blood sugar may fall rapidly, because of an imbalance between insulin and sugar — i.e. too much insulin and not enough sugar in the blood — the body responds and will return the blood sugar to normal. It does this in two ways, firstly by breaking down body stores of starch, and secondly by producing a substance called glucagon. Why, then, does the hypoglycaemic reaction occur? The answer is quite simply that the body's response is not fast enough. However, it will catch up eventually, and the child will recover, even if no sugar has been given. Thus, there is no reason why you should worry unduly about hypoglycaemia, and certainly there is no need to set up a night rota so that your child is constantly watched over.

Insulin reaction and convulsions

Occasionally, because of the rapid lowering of blood sugar during an insulin reaction, the brain may respond by producing a convulsion (commonly called a 'fit'). This is one of the most frightening aspects of an insulin reaction. However, if you have experienced someone suffering a convulsion, you will know that the effects appear much more alarming than they really are.

What should you do if your child develops a convulsion? The first point to stress is that if your child is unconscious or having a fit, you should not try to get him or her to take anything by mouth. In any case, this may be virtually impossible to do, since the teeth may be tightly clenched. Within a few minutes, however, the body will start to produce sugar from its own stores, the blood sugar will rise and your child will recover.

Treatment of severe reactions

Obviously, severe reactions are best avoided whenever possible, but if they should occur, they can be dealt with by means of a simple injection of glucagon, which is a natural substance produced by the body in its attempt to stem the reaction.

Glucagon is available on prescription, in the form of a simple kit. It should be injected either under the skin or into a muscle (see Appendix 4, page 201). Within a few minutes the unconscious child should recover — but as the effect of glucagon is only temporary you must <u>always</u> give some sugar once consciousness has been regained. If recovery does not occur, then you should call a doctor immediately.

Here is a summary of the steps you must take if your child has a convulsion or is deeply unconscious:

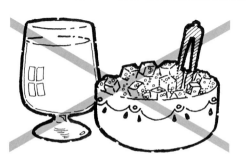

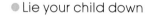

- Lie your child down

- Keep him/her warm

- <u>Do not</u> try to give sugar or sugar fluid

● Give an injection of glucagon
(details in Appendix 4)

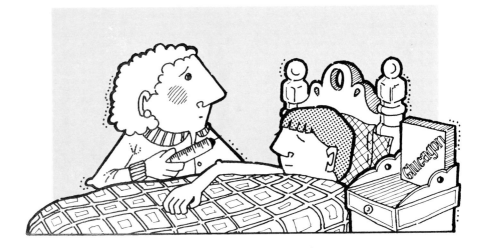

● Once recovery takes place, give a glass of
water or juice with four teaspoonsful of sugar

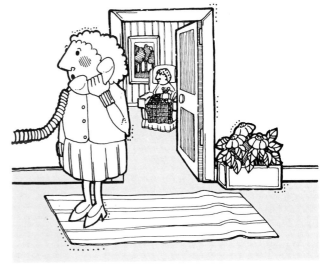

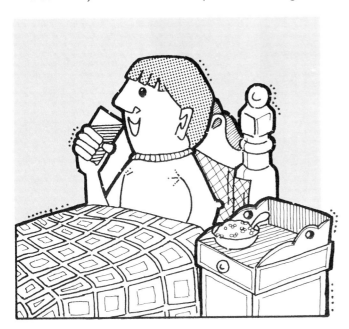

● If recovery does not occur, or if this is the first time
your child has had a convulsion, call your
doctor who, if your child is still unconscious
when he arrives, will probably administer
glucose into a vein.

Is it a reaction?

When your child looks peaky or is unwell, you may be concerned that it could be a symptom of an insulin reaction. A headache may be an indication of hypoglycaemia, especially if it occurs in the early morning. Variation in mood is also sometimes attributed to a low blood sugar, but if this is the case it should not last long and will rapidly improve with sugar. In most cases where these 'symptoms' occur your child will not be hypoglycaemic — but, of course, you will want to be sure. In time, you will get to know the pattern of your child's reactions, and this knowledge, combined with an understanding of the usual symptoms of hypoglycaemia (see Chapter 6, page 88), will help you to decide. With small children, in particular, whose behaviour and health wax and wane with remarkable speed, you may find it especially difficult to decide whether your child is suffering an impending reaction, or is merely tired, hungry, or fed up. The only foolproof way of finding out is to perform one of the blood tests (see Appendix 3, page 197).

Understandably, you will not want to perform blood tests every time your child is below par. The best guide as to what you should do is provided by the frequency of the episodes. Thus, if they are occurring at a time when you would expect your child to be hungry or short of sugar, give him or her something to eat. The only times you need have any concern are if these episodes happen very frequently and you are constantly having to provide a lot of extra carbohydrate, or if your child is getting fat.

You should beware of the fact that most children will quickly realise that if they say they "feel funny", they may get a Mars bar — and who would not exploit this possibility!

If blood tests show the blood sugar to be within the normal range when these episodes occur, then your child is not suffering a hypoglycaemic reaction.

Intelligence and hypoglycaemic reactions

Many parents worry that episodes of hypoglycaemia, especially if associated with bouts of unconsciousness or convulsions, may lead to deterioration in the intelligence and development of their child. Such fears are groundless, and the growth and mental development of a child who is reasonably well controlled will be normal, even if fairly frequent reactions occur.

Too much . . . too little

If your child seems constantly hungry, then it would be appropriate, as with any other child, to give him or her more to eat. Unless you are sure that the hunger is due to a reaction, any additional food should be given at normal meal and snack times. If your child is of normal weight, there is no harm in increasing the amount of food, but if your child is overweight or fat, then some care is necessary in giving anything extra.

Never reduce the recommended diet

IMPORTANT: if the tests are all positive you must NEVER try to improve your child's diabetic control by cutting down on food or cutting out normal meals.

Should your child be getting an illicit supply of sugar, in the form of sweets or sweet drinks, this ought to be prevented, but your child's normal diet should not be reduced in an attempt to improve the results of the tests. If the tests are positive with a normal diet, your child needs more insulin, not less food.

Parties

As far as possible, your child's social activities should continue as normal. With smaller children you may worry about what they might eat when not under your supervision. A word with the person in charge will guard against too much sugar or sweet food being eaten. Even so, the worst that might happen is a rise in tests for a day or two, but this will do no harm.

You may be concerned about the timing of the tea-time insulin injection. If the party is during the afternoon, it is probably best to give the injection when your child comes home, with a top-up snack before bedtime. If the party is prolonged into the evening, then it is best to give the injection before the meal, if it is not too complicated to arrange. More information on parties and discos is given in Chapter 9, page 132.

Problems with tests

Small children and testing

With very small children and infants, testing may be a problem. Once your child is potty trained, urine testing is straightforward, using the technique described in Appendix 2, page 189. Problems can arise, however, with a child who is still in nappies, although simply squeezing a little urine from a wet nappy onto a testing strip may be adequate. If you find that this form of testing is problematical, then an occasional blood test will reassure you that all is well.

With all children, but especially the younger ones, it is difficult to get them to urinate at exactly the time you need to perform a test. In such cases, just make a note of the times that urine is passed and your doctor can then help you to interpret the results of these tests, so that you can make any necessary adjustments to your child's diet or insulin dose.

Why must I be tested?

This question is often asked by children. Although many youngsters can appreciate the reasons for testing, the very young cannot be expected to understand what is being done or why. Even so, most children become so accustomed to tests, that they view them in much the same way as any of their other routines, such as toothbrushing and washing. Young children question the reasons less frequently than older children, who often do not want to accept the inconvenience of what they consider to be a boring routine.

Frequently, older children may practise all sorts of ploys to avoid tests: "My tests were all normal, so I haven't written them down"; or "I forgot"; or "I threw it (the urine) away by mistake". In dealing with this situation bribery is unwise. You should adopt a consistent approach in which you reinforce the message that tests are essential if treatment is to be balanced and health and fitness maintained.

More insulin

When tests are consistently high, <u>more</u> insulin is required. At such times, parents frequently ask, "Can I adjust the insulin dose myself?". The answer to this question is "Yes". In fact, adjustment of insulin should be the rule, rather than the exception. Of course, during the early stages you will need advice from your doctor, specialist nurse or diabetes health visitor as to when and by how much the insulin dose should be increased. There are no set rules, because the dose required by each child is different. More insulin is often required when your child is less active, for example when at home for the weekend, or on holiday, or during any of the childhood illnesses.

Less insulin

If your child suffers frequent reactions (they usually occur at approximately the same time of day), less insulin may be needed.

Giving less insulin is preferable to attempting to counter persistent reactions by giving excess glucose or sweet things. By getting to know how long the effect of each insulin dose lasts, you should be able to work out which dose or type of insulin should be reduced and by how much.

Children often require less insulin when they are at school, since at such times they may be more active and consequently their blood sugar is lower.

Initially, adjusting the insulin dose will undoubtedly seem frighteningly complicated, but with practice and guidance from doctors or diabetes specialist nurses you will soon become quite capable of making the necessary adjustments. It all boils down to plain common sense:

- The child with a <u>high</u> blood sugar needs <u>more</u> insulin.

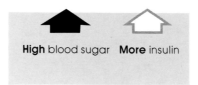

- The child with a <u>low</u> blood sugar needs <u>less</u> insulin or <u>more</u> food.

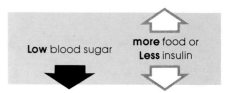

As for making a major error and causing damage to your child, if you make the sort of adjustments you have been advised, then the risks are negligible.

When you have to be away from your child

There will be occasions when you wish to leave your child in the care of somebody else. A close relative will probably be aware of how to take care of your child, but a babysitter will need some simple instructions. An example of a suitable chart (available from the British Diabetic Association) is given in Appendix 8, page 227.

SCHOOL AND DIABETES

Telling the teacher

It is important that all the teachers are aware that your child has diabetes, for two reasons:

1 Mid-morning or afternoon snacks must be permitted and, particularly in the case of young children, the teachers can help to ensure that these and main meals are taken on time and not missed.

2 The teachers should understand what is happening if your child should have a hypoglycaemic reaction. Teachers should be told how to treat these reactions, and should be discouraged from sending your child home, when giving a biscuit or two or three lumps of sugar is sufficient to curtail most reactions.

Unnecessary fear of reactions and over-protective attitudes will be prevented by having discussions with the teachers as soon as your child starts school, or when diabetes is first diagnosed. Also, you should give them a copy of the special leaflet for teachers (see Appendix 7, page 225), available from the British Diabetic Association. Your doctor or specialist nurse will be happy to talk to them.

School meals

Parents often worry about the quality and quantity of school meals. The choice lies between school dinners, packed lunches, and coming home for lunch. It is important that your child should do as other children do, and not be made to feel or appear different in any way.

School meals usually contain adequate amounts of carbohydrate to provide the correct portions. You should not be over-concerned that mistakes may be made which will upset your child's diabetic control. If the school operates a cafeteria system, it may be more difficult for your child to select the right type of food. If your child is very young, you can check through the school menus, and ask the teacher concerned to help with the right choice of food.

The decision as to whether or not your child should have school meals should not be influenced by your child's diabetes. Only if control becomes difficult should you consider providing a packed lunch or lunch at home.

Exercise

At school, the timing and extent of exercise can usually be determined in advance and any difficulties anticipated. Below, we answer some of the questions parents most commonly ask about exercise.

Do I need to give my child extra carbohydrate before exercise?
Yes. It is essential that games teachers appreciate the importance of this extra carbohydrate, and ensure that your child takes it before any exercise.

Fig. 10.3
Exercise and sport are essential for all children with diabetes.
Photos: Chris Schwarz.

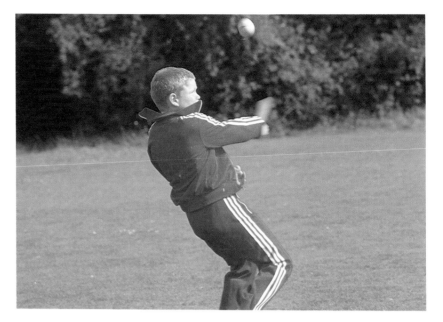

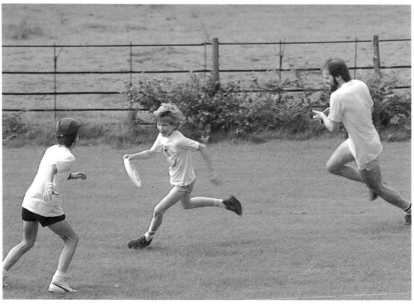

Are there any activities or sports in which my child should not participate?

No, having diabetes is no bar to participating in any normal sporting activity, and it should not be used as an excuse for missing games. Very high levels of achievement have been reached in many sports, by those with diabetes.

Older children may wish to take part in more dangerous sports, such as climbing or sailing, and these activities need to be given more careful consideration. It is essential that your child should be accompanied, and that hypoglycaemic reactions are prevented.

What if my child becomes hypoglycaemic during exercise?

Your child should take more sugar. Make sure the teachers in charge know exactly what to do.

Should I be present during games periods?

No. You should resist any pressure which might be exerted to persuade you to be present, since this would merely serve to single out your child as being 'different'.

My child is putting on weight and would appear to require large quantities of extra carbohydrate in order to avoid hypoglycaemia during exercise — what should I do?

The best advice is to reduce the insulin dosage, rather than continue to increase the carbohydrate intake. This should be done on the days when heavy exercise is likely, with a return to the normal insulin dosage on other days.

How should I deal with unexpected periods of exercise, say at weekends?

On most occasions an extra portion or two of carbohydrate will be sufficient to guard against any risk of reactions.

I get very worried when my child goes off to play alone or with friends at the local recreation ground — should I take any special precautions?

This is a cause for concern for many parents. The guiding principle should be that you provide the same supervision for a child with diabetes as you would for any child of the same age. If your child has a mishap, whether it be a broken ankle or a hypoglycaemic reaction, friends will always summon aid, so don't worry unduly!

The effect of stress on diabetes

One of the commonest reasons for an increase in blood sugar is anxiety. All children are stressed at times; it may be minor worries about losing something, or failing to complete work to the teacher's satisfaction. In those without diabetes, these stresses may go unnoticed, but with diabetes it may result in positive urine tests, or blood tests which show high levels of blood sugar. If you are perplexed by inexplicable changes in the control pattern, stress could well be the answer.

Occasionally, severe stress may be associated with hypoglycaemia, but this is less common.

Urine testing at school

It is clearly awkward for children to perform urine tests at school. The lavatories are often unsocial places to do this, and most children feel uncomfortable at the prospect. Therefore, it is often recommended that mid-day tests at school need not be done unless difficulties arise with your child's control. At such times, the 'dipstick' procedures are easier. If your child finds performing urine tests too embarrassing, blood tests may be preferred.

School attendance and performance

School attendance should be the same as that for any other child. In general, it is found that children with diabetes are not significantly more absent from school than their non-diabetic counterparts.

Your child's intellectual, sporting and general activities should also be similar to those of other children.

Staying away, holidays and travel

Children with diabetes should be encouraged to participate in all those activities which would be expected of other children. These include nights or weekends away, camps of various kinds, travel at home and overseas. Certainly, you should not discourage your child from going on holiday either in this country or abroad.

Nights and weekends away

All parents are apprehensive the first time their children stay away from home, but as the parent of a child with diabetes, you will probably feel particularly concerned. Before your child stays away, you should be sure of two facts, namely, that:

1. Your child is capable of giving his or her own injections, or there is an adult present who can give them.

2. The people with whom your child will be staying are fully aware of the possibility of hypoglycaemic reactions, and know what to do should they face one. It is important that you should not be afraid to ask them to:

   - Be particularly attentive to any changes in your child's moods or health

   - Make sure the diet does not contain excessively sweet food

   - Check that insulin is taken at the correct dosage and at the set times.

You will find that most responsible people will be only too willing to help in any way possible.

Whenever you feel anxious, always remind yourself that even untreated children will recover from reactions.

Camps

Cub camps, brownie weekends and brigade camps are important childhood activities. They are always well supervised by people with first aid experience, and as long as you inform them about your child's diabetes, you may be confident that all will be well.

For children worried by the prospect of going away from home, the British Diabetic Association's educational holidays perform a very important function, enabling them to enjoy a holiday in a situation where they need not feel the 'odd men out'. Because the camps are well supervised by specialist staff, you should be able to feel at ease in the knowledge that your child is being provided with the best possible care. For more information, contact the British Diabetic Association.

Fig. 10.4
Children with diabetes can participate in all the usual childhood activities, including holidays abroad, adventure holidays and camps.

Photo: Chris Schwarz.

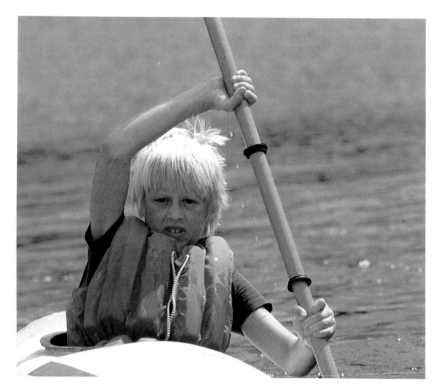

Effects of travel

Overseas travel should pose no particular problems. Your experience of selecting the right sort of food for your child when at home will enable you to select from even the most unusual foreign menus. The worst that can happen is that the blood sugar level goes a little higher than normal.

Travel sickness

The actual journeys should pose little difficulty, apart from travel sickness (see also Chapter 9, page 126). Although this is relatively common, you may worry that vomiting may lead to diabetic ketosis (see Chapter 6, page 81). Fortunately, travel sickness is confined to the period of travel, and as soon as the motion ceases, so does the nausea and vomiting. With long car journeys, break the journey frequently, avoid reading and, if necessary, try to obtain some motion sickness tablets from your doctor. Should your child be sick, give sweetened juices every hour to ensure that loss of fluid and fat breakdown do not occur. If you are on a long journey, say by sea, you may find that the tests become positive, in which case an increase in insulin dose may be necessary.

Meal times

Most children find journeys exciting, and hence it is likely that the blood sugar will rise. Therefore, hypoglycaemic reactions during long journeys are most unlikely, and you should keep snacks and meals to normal times. Increasing the food intake should not be necessary, but it is a wise precaution to carry some extra snacks, in case meals should be unduly delayed.

Air travel

Air travel can be a little difficult due to time changes. This subject is discussed in more detail in Chapter 9, page 129.

Insurance

When travelling abroad you should always make sure that you

have some health insurance (see Chapter 9, page 129), and in an EEC country you should have the appropriate forms for free treatment (Form E111), available from your local DSS office.

Vaccination and immunization

Vaccinations and immunizations can be given to your child in exactly the same way as for any other child. The worst that can happen with some types of vaccination, such as TAB, is that your child may feel slightly unwell for twenty four hours or so, and that the blood sugar may rise. If the tests become positive, you may need to increase the dose of insulin, just as you would with any other minor illness.

Sickness while away

Short vomiting illnesses are quite common. When travelling, these should be managed in exactly the same way as any other illness, and you should refer to Chapter 9, page 128 and this chapter, page 161. Familiarize yourself with these sections before you go on holiday.

OLDER CHILDREN WITH DIABETES

Teaching your children about diabetes

The earlier children take an active interest in their diabetes, particularly in giving their own injections, the better. In the early stages in younger children, detailed explanations are unlikely to be fully understood. However, as children grow older, it will be necessary for them to take complete command of their treatment, so that they can achieve the independence they seek. Their success depends, to a large extent, on you. Your child will need to learn as much about diabetes as you know, and be persuaded that the steps necessary to maintain good balance are worthwhile, because they ensure a fit, healthy, active life. During adolescence, special counselling sessions may be arranged for your child, either alone or in your presence. These can be of real value in providing answers to questions which you may not be able to answer adequately. They also serve the important function of reinforcing what you, Mum or Dad, might have said — and, as you will be only too aware, what Mum or Dad says is not always listened to!

Ignoring diabetes

Most parents find that the adolescent may be more concerned about things other than their diabetes! They find the whole subject of diabetes boring, and the non-stop treatment tedious. As a result, fewer tests may be performed, a degree of sloppiness may creep into insulin technique and the timing of doses. A lax attitude may develop with regard to the regularity of meals and the type of food eaten. It is as well for you to be prepared for this, otherwise it can cause considerable frustration and anger. Try to appreciate that your child will be seeing himself or herself as an individual for the first time — an image that is marred by a total dependence on the daily injection of insulin. At a time when striving for independence is the main goal, many adolescents find this intolerable, and occasional displays of anger and rejection are hardly surprising. This period of rejection is, however, usually short-lived. It is important for you to remind yourself during this difficult time that short periods of loss of control — weeks or even a month or two — will not be serious in terms of its influence on long-term complications. Remain confident that your son or daughter will return to a more responsible approach to diabetes, and make every effort to:

- Try to be understanding
- Treat your son or daughter as an adult rather than a child
- Encourage an attitude of responsibility with regard to treatment and clinic attendance
- Stay cool!

Manipulation

Young people frequently develop ways of ensuring that their diabetes gives rise to as little inconvenience as possible. They work out that negative urine tests are always approved of, and they may decide that the easiest way of achieving this is not to test at all, but simply to write down the desired results. Your doctor may perceive what is happening, but if he does not and you do, you should tell him, so that he can make sure that your child is getting the correct dose of insulin.

Children who have severe anxieties about their diabetes, or those who feel very insecure, may occasionally manipulate things in a more extreme and possibly risky way. For example, in an effort to get attention, they may even manipulate their insulin injections or meals so that reactions occur more frequently. This, of course, creates a good deal of concern from both parents and doctors, and may lead to admission to hospital, where the child will feel more secure. If your child shows signs of behaving in this disturbing way, you should seek expert help. You should not automatically feel that you are failing in some way to provide the care and support that your child needs. Also, you should remember that it is sometimes very difficult for children to express their fears about their health to anyone, perhaps least of all to their parents, whose esteem they treasure most highly. Sometimes, by causing reactions, they hope to get the help and attention of a third party, such as the doctor or specialist nurse, with whom they may be able to discuss their problems more readily.

Teenage activities

As your child grows up, his or her activities will become very much more varied, and some routines which were once easy often become more difficult to maintain. Therefore, it is important that diabetes should impose as few restrictions as possible on day-to-day activities. A twice-daily dosage of insulin provides considerable flexibility with regard to injection times, thereby enabling the time of, say, the evening meal, to be changed in order to permit participation in after-school activities. If the evening meal is delayed by more than half an hour, a small snack should be eaten to cover any residual effects of the early morning insulin dose. The evening dose of insulin should then be given before the main meal.

One other aspect of teenage life which may worry you is that your child might eat the wrong sort of food and drink sucrose-containing drinks when at parties or discos. If this happens it is not going to cause any major problems, so don't worry unnecessarily (more advice about parties and discos is given in Chapter 9, page 132). It is vital that your child should not be constantly precluded from normal teenage activities, simply because of his or her diabetes.

CHILDREN WITH DIABETES AND OTHER ILLNESSES

The effect of diabetes on other illnesses and their treatment

Many parents are concerned that diabetes may lead to increased frequency of other illnesses. The fears are, in the main, groundless, and your child should be no more prone to catching coughs, colds and childhood infections, such as chickenpox, than any other child.

A child with diabetes can undergo all forms of treatment. With operations, however, one or two special precautions will need to be taken. For example, if the operation is likely to lead to a long period during which your child is unable to eat, then a drip or intravenous feeding may be necessary.

Dentistry

Some precautions are necessary to maintain diabetic balance during treatment. Further details are provided in Chapter 7, page 104.

Can other illnesses affect your child's diabetes?

Yes, any illness will tend to raise the blood sugar, requiring an increase in the insulin dose.

Particular care is required with illnesses associated with:

- Vomiting
- Nausea
- Loss of appetite.

These are far more common in children than in adults, and vomiting, in particular, can be associated with almost any illness. The standard procedures to be followed in cases of vomiting are described in Chapter 6, page 82, and they should be carefully adhered to if the risk of the serious complication of diabetic keto-acidosis is to be avoided. Because these procedures are so important, they are summarized below.

If meals are omitted due to loss of appetite or vomiting, you must do as follows:

 Never reduce or stop insulin.

 Test the urine or blood. If the urine is negative for sugar, or blood tests show the blood sugar to be within the normal range, continue with the normal dose of insulin.

 If there is a large amount of sugar in the urine, or the blood sugar is very high, increase the dose of insulin by the amounts recommended by your doctor. Therefore, it is essential that you check these amounts with your doctor before your child is sick.

 Replace the portions of meals and snacks by hourly drinks containing sugar, at the rate of one good-sized glassful every hour. These drinks can be fruit juices, Lucozade, or other sweetened drinks, such as Coca Cola.

 Continue to test the urine or blood, and give sweetened drinks until your child is eating normally again.

 If your doctor considers it necessary, give an additional dose of short-acting insulin.

 Vomiting, nausea or loss of appetite usually last only a relatively short time, so if your child fails to improve within a few hours, consult your doctor or diabetic clinic.

DIABETES AND YOUR OTHER CHILDREN

Inheritance

If you have other children, or you intend having more in the future, you might well be concerned that they, too, could develop diabetes. The risk of insulin dependent diabetes being inherited is small (see Chapter 8, page 109). In fact, the type of diabetes most commonly inherited is non-insulin dependent diabetes. On the whole, it is recommended that you should plan the family you want and not be put off by the fear of another child having diabetes. If at any time you are worried that one of your children has symptoms of diabetes, you can readily put your mind at rest by performing a blood or urine test.

Reactions of your other children to your diabetic child

One of the problems which you are likely to encounter is that your child with diabetes may be seen by any brothers or sisters to be receiving more attention than themselves. This may lead to misunderstandings and it is wise, therefore, to remind your other children of the disadvantages and difficulties of having diabetes.

A topic which you must discuss with your other children is the problem of hypoglycaemia and how to deal with it. They should be taught to give sugar during a reaction, and to make sure that an adult is told. Severe hypoglycaemic reactions, especially if associated with a fit, can be very alarming to a small brother or sister, but if they are forewarned then it may not be so frightening.

Diabetes and the family diet

Many parents are surprised to learn that the diet for diabetes is really a rather good one. Such a diet contains very little sugar, which damages the teeth, and sufficient carbohydrate, protein and fat to ensure full growth and development, but not so much that it causes obesity. Your family may react strongly at first to any reduction in sweet food and drinks, but it is surprising how quickly children, in particular, can develop a taste for savoury food. Older members of the family, with long-established eating habits, will probably be the most resistant to change, even though they may appreciate the possible benefits of a healthier diet.

Of course, apart from the health aspect, the fact that the whole family eats a diabetic-type diet always makes life a lot easier for the cook!

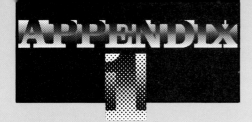
HOW TO INJECT INSULIN

This section summarizes the techniques that are used, <u>but you must be shown how to inject before doing so yourself.</u>

Equipment required

Fig. A1.1
Essential equipment for injecting insulin.

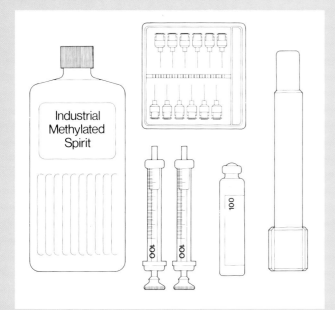

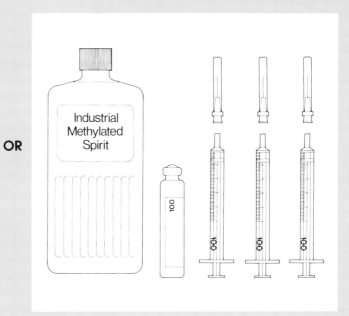

OR

- Insulin
- At least two glass syringes and a supply of needles.
- A carrying case
- Industrial spirit

- Insulin
- A supply of disposable syringes and disposable needles.
- Industrial spirit

Syringes and needles

Two types of syringe are available:

1. Glass syringes with separate needles, which may be stainless steel or disposable.
2. Plastic disposable syringes with built-in or separate disposable needles.

All syringes are available in two sizes (Fig. A1.2); 0.5ml (showing 50 units, each division representing 1 unit) and 1ml (showing 100 units, each division representing 2 units).

Fig. A1.2
Syringes are available in two sizes.

½ml syringe (50 units)
1 division = 1 unit

1ml syringe (100 units)
1 division = 2 units

THE NUMBER OF UNITS YOU DRAW UP
=THE NUMBER OF UNITS IN YOUR DOSE

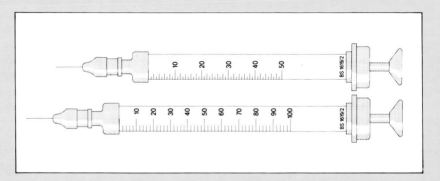

How to draw up your insulin

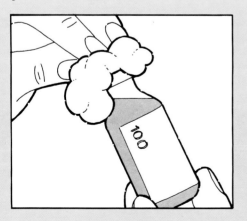

Using one type of insulin from one bottle only

1. Clean the rubber cap of the bottle with industrial spirit.

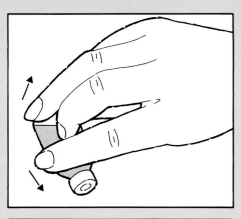

2. Turn the bottle upside down a few times to make sure that the insulin is thoroughly mixed.

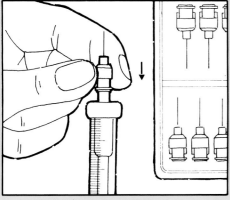

3. Remove the needle from its container and fix securely onto the syringe (or remove cap from disposable syringe).

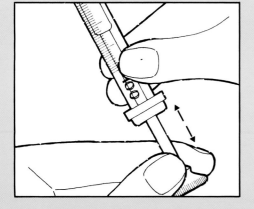

4. Work the syringe plunger in and out a few times to make sure that it moves freely and that any fluid still in it is expelled.

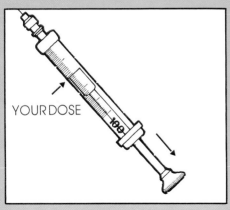

YOUR DOSE

5. Pull out the plunger to the exact number of units of your dose, in order to draw air into the syringe.

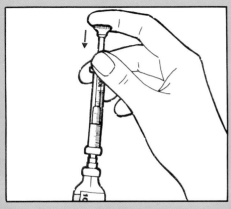

6. Insert the needle straight through the rubber cap of the insulin bottle and push in the plunger of the syringe to inject all of the air into the bottle.

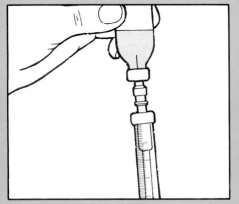

7. Turn the bottle upside down, making sure that the needle point is well below the surface level of the insulin in the bottle.

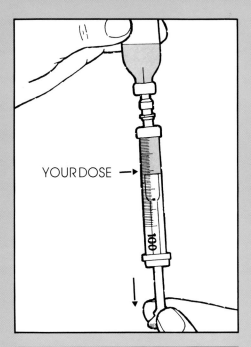

YOUR DOSE →

8. Holding the bottle in the same position, pull out the plunger, which will suck the insulin into the syringe, until you have drawn up slightly more insulin than you need.

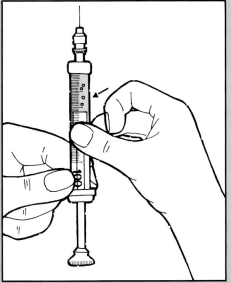

9. Pull the needle out of the bottle and, still holding the syringe with the needle pointing upwards, tap the syringe gently to allow any air bubbles to rise to the top. If the bubbles persist, re-insert the needle into the bottle, push out the insulin from the syringe and start again from Step 7.

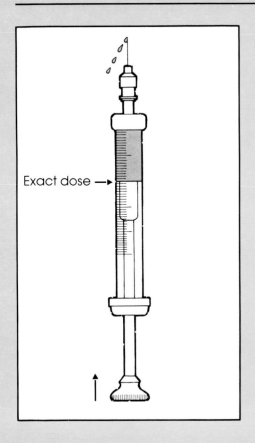

Exact dose →

10. Push in the plunger to expel unwanted air and excess insulin, until the top of the plunger is level with the number of units on the syringe equal to your dose of insulin.

Using a mixture of two types of insulin (clear and cloudy)

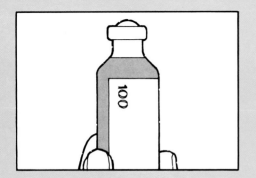

1. Check the insulin bottles.

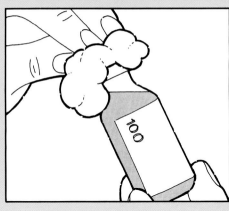

2. Clean the rubber caps of the bottles with industrial spirit.

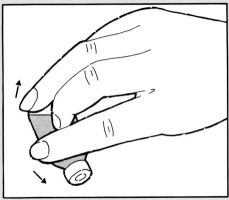

3. Turn the bottles upside down a few times to make sure that the insulins are thoroughly mixed.

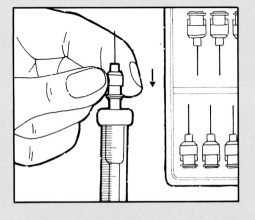

4. Remove the needle from its container and fix securely onto the syringe.

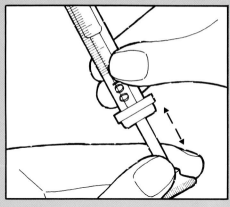

5. Work the plunger in and out a few times to make sure that it moves freely and that any fluid still in it is expelled.

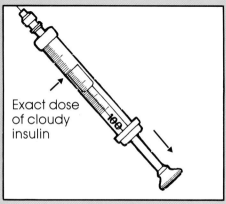

Exact dose of cloudy insulin

6. Pull out the plunger to the <u>exact number of units of your dose of cloudy insulin,</u> in order to draw air into the syringe.

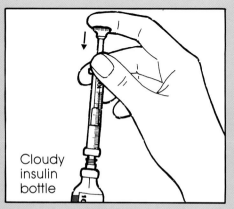

Cloudy insulin bottle

7. With the bottle of <u>cloudy</u> insulin held upright, insert the needle straight down through the rubber cap of the cloudy insulin bottle. Keeping the point of the needle above the level of the insulin in the bottle, push in the plunger of the syringe to inject air into the bottle.

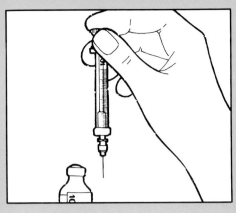

8. Pull out the syringe and needle, keeping the plunger pushed in.

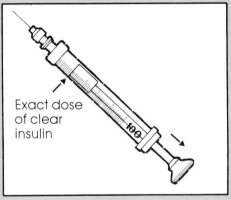

Exact dose of clear insulin

9. Work the plunger in and out a few times to check that it is still free, and then pull out the plunger to the exact number of units of your dose of clear insulin, in order to draw air into the syringe.

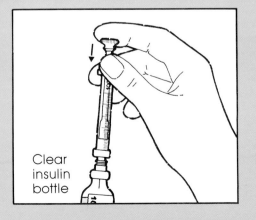

Clear insulin bottle

10. Insert the needle straight through the rubber cap of the clear insulin bottle and push in the plunger of the syringe to inject air into the bottle.

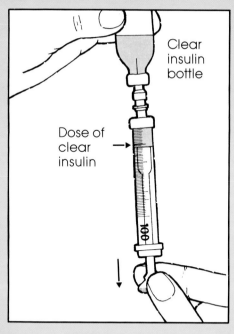

Clear
insulin
bottle

Dose of
clear
insulin →

11. Turn the bottle upside down, making sure the needle point is well below the surface level of the clear insulin.

12. Holding the bottle in the same position, pull out the plunger, which will suck the clear insulin into the syringe, until you have slightly more clear insulin than you need.

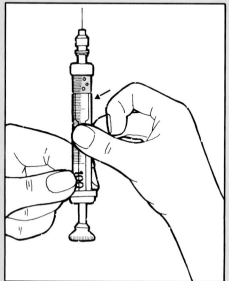

13. Pull the needle out of the bottle and, still holding the syringe with the needle pointing upwards, tap the syringe gently to allow any air bubbles to rise to the top. If the bubbles persist, re-insert the needle into the bottle and start again from step 11.

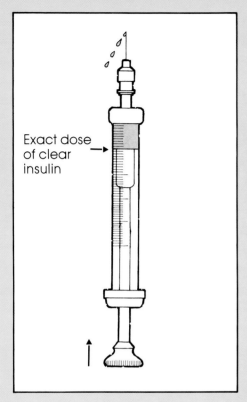

Exact dose of clear insulin

14. Expel unwanted air and excess clear insulin by pushing in the plunger. The top of the plunger should be level with the number of units on the syringe barrel equal to your exact dose of clear insulin.

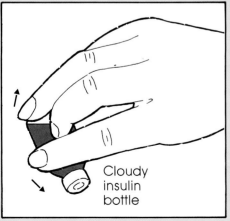

Cloudy insulin bottle

15. Now take the bottle of <u>cloudy</u> insulin and, once again, tip it upside down a couple of times.

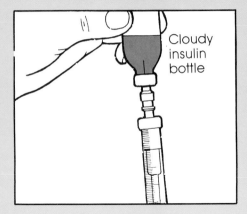

Cloudy insulin bottle

16. Holding the _cloudy_ insulin bottle upside down, insert the needle through the rubber cap of the bottle, making certain that the point of the needle is well below the surface of the insulin.

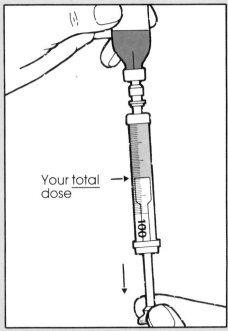

Your <u>total</u> dose →

17. Holding the bottle upside down, draw up the insulin into the syringe by pulling out the plunger from its original position (the position equal to the number of units of clear insulin), so that the top of the plunger is now level with the number of units on the syringe equal to your exact dose of cloudy insulin. It is important to note that <u>the final position of the plunger will be at a point equal to the total dose of clear plus cloudy insulin.</u>
Withdraw the needle from the cloudy bottle.

Dose of clear insulin ⌐ Dose of cloudy insulin

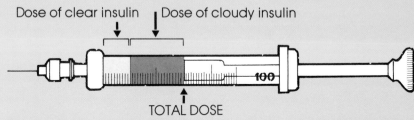

TOTAL DOSE

There are two important points to remember when using two-dose injections:

1. <u>Always draw up the clear insulin into the syringe first.</u>

2. <u>If you should accidentally draw up too much cloudy insulin, do not push it back into the cloudy insulin bottle, since this will introduce a mixture of clear and cloudy insulin into the cloudy bottle. The safest procedure is to discard all the insulin in the syringe and start again from step 4.</u>

Injecting insulin

Having drawn up the insulin into the syringe, you are now ready to inject it. You can choose any of the injection sites shown in Fig. A1.3. You should use one site for the morning injection and a different site for the evening injection, e.g. arms in the morning, legs in the evening; but vary the side, e.g. left on Monday, right on Tuesday, etc. Having chosen a general area, you should make sure that you vary the point of entry each day. If this is not done you will develop a scar, which will prevent the insulin from being adequately absorbed.

Fig. A1.3
Where to inject insulin.

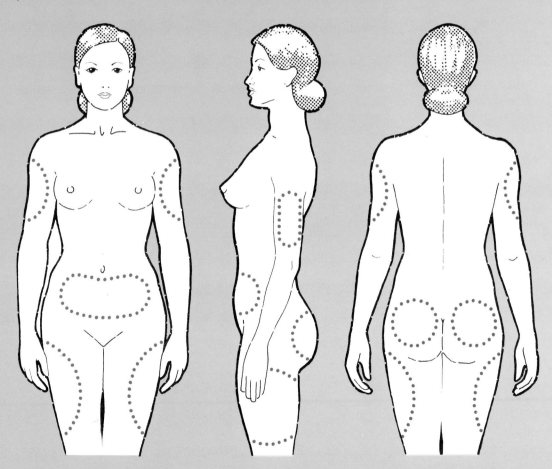

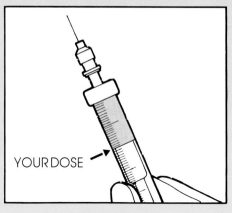

YOUR DOSE

Method

1. Check that you have drawn up the correct amount of insulin.

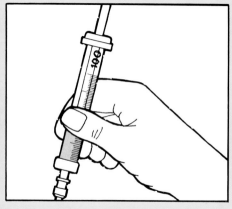

2. Without touching the sterile tip of the needle, hold the syringe as shown.

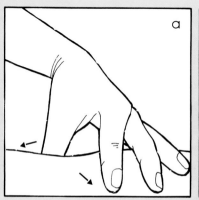

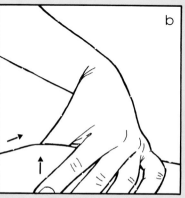

3. If there is ample flesh at the injection site, stretch flat an area of clean skin between the thumb and forefinger (a). If there is little flesh at the injection site, pinch up a mound of skin between thumb and forefinger (b).

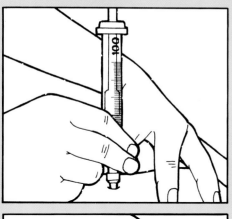

4. Push the needle straight into the flat area of the skin, as quickly as you can. The depth to which you push the needle will depend on the size needle you use. With a short needle (less than ½ inch) push it in to the hilt; with a larger needle push it in about half of its length.

The needle <u>must penetrate below the skin</u>, otherwise you may produce blisters shortly after the injection. On the other hand, if the injection is too deep, it may be painful.

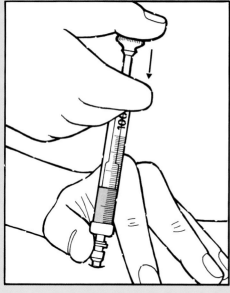

5. Holding the syringe in one hand, press in the plunger smoothly and quicky.

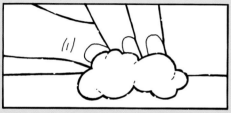

6. Pull out the needle and place a clean piece of cotton wool, swab or tissue over the needle mark, holding it in position for a few seconds.

Equipment for multiple injections

Devices are now available to enable you to give multiple injections of insulin, and to enable you to carry sufficient insulin for your daily requirements.

Fig. A1.4
The Penject for multiple injections of insulin.

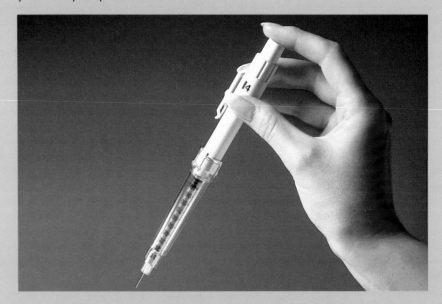

Injector guns

Another method of injecting insulin involves the use of triggered injecting equipment, known as an injector gun. Unfortunately, the gun has numerous disadvantages: it is cumbersome and therefore not easily carried; siting injections can be difficult; and, surprisingly, it can sometimes be more painful than injecting with a glass or disposable syringe.

Problems with injections

Fear of giving injections

After giving your first injection, much of the fear will disappear. Like most people with diabetes, you will no doubt have been surprised that the injection was almost painless.

Spilling insulin

If insulin squirts out from around the needle when you press in the plunger, do not worry. It is important that you should not start all over again, unless you are sure that all the insulin has been wasted in this way. Rather than worry about whether you have taken in sufficient insulin, it is better and safer to pay particular attention to your test results. One faulty injection will not have serious consequences.

Swelling and pain at the injection site

It is quite common for a little redness to develop at the site of the injection. This may persist for a day or two when you first start injections, but it usually disappears after a week or so.

Occasionally, you may develop little blisters when you inject, usually because you are not injecting deeply enough. If after injecting more deeply you still develop blisters, tell your doctor.

Infection at the injection site

Infection of this nature is very rare. With reasonable cleanliness — you don't need a gown and gloves — this should never occur.

Some commonly asked questions about injections

Because injections are such a common cause for concern, it may prove useful to answer a few of the most frequently asked questions.

Will the needle cause damage if I'm clumsy?

No. If you inject where you are shown to inject, you cannot do any damage.

Do I have to clean the skin with spirit?

No, this merely hardens the skin. Providing that the skin is clean, no swabbing with spirit is necessary.

Can I be allergic to insulin?

This occurs very rarely and will be obvious to your doctor at the outset. If you are allergic, the problem can be readily overcome by changing to another type of insulin.

What if I can't see to measure the insulin?

If you have poor eyesight, it is still possible to draw up insulin and give your own injection by using special pre-set or click count syringes (Fig. A1.5a).

Another aid which you might find helpful is a magnifying glass which clips onto glass or disposable syringes (Fig. A1.5b).

Fig. A1.5
Aids for those with poor sight.

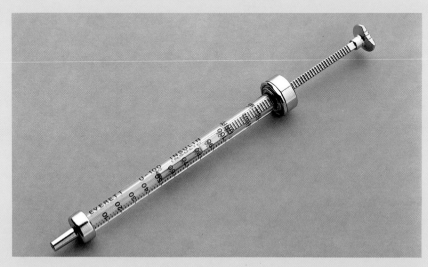

a. Click-count syringe

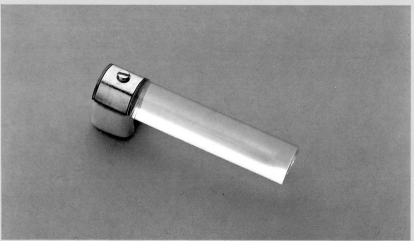

b. Magnifying glass

Care of your syringe

Glass syringe and re-usable needle

Draw up a little spirit into your syringe and rinse it out. Put the syringe and needle into your carrying case or other container, which should be half-filled with spirit. It is not necessary to boil your syringe.

Disposable needles

Although intended to be used only once, most people find that they can use them several times before they get blunt.

Disposable syringes

Like disposable needles, these are intended to be used once only. It is quite safe to use these syringes more than once, however, providing the markings do not become so worn that it is difficult to measure the dose accurately.

If you decide to use a disposable syringe more than once, then after each injection you should leave a needle on the end, cover it with its sterile cap, and keep it in a refrigerator. If the syringe has a built-in needle, just replace the needle cap after use.

Occasionally, needles become blocked, especially very fine ones, such as BD-Plastipak. To check for a blockage, work the plunger in and out and if resistance is felt or if it is very difficult to draw up the insulin, discard the needle and use another.

There are two important points to remember when using a disposable syringe:

1. Never put it in spirit.
2. If the markings are at all indistinct, use a new syringe.

Disposal of used syringes and needles

Disposable syringes

Break off the needle and then place the needle and syringe in an empty beer or Coke can. When the can is full, seal up the hole, and put it in the dustbin.

Disposable syringes can be burned if a suitable incinerator is available.

Glass syringes

Wrap the syringe in newspaper, and hit the syringe with a hammer or other suitably heavy object, in order to break the glass. Place the wrapped syringe in the dustbin.

Used needles

Collect needles in an empty beer or Coke can until full. After sealing the hole, place the can in the dustbin.

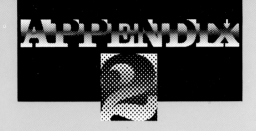
URINE TESTS

There are three reliable tests available in this country — Clinitest, Diabur-Test 5000 and Diastix (Fig. 4.7, page 70). Clinitest is slightly more sensitive and the colour change is easier to observe, but it does have the disadvantage that it requires the collection of a specimen of urine to put in a tube for testing. Diabur-Test 5000 and Diastix have the advantage that they are simpler to use, but if your sight is not perfect they may be less accurate.

There is a fourth test available, Clinistix, but this is not recommended, because it only tells you whether sugar is present or absent.

When interpreting the results of your urine tests, it is important to know when you last passed urine. If you passed urine half an hour before doing the test, then the amount of sugar in the urine will represent the level of sugar in the blood during the half hour before testing. If, however, you have not passed urine for several hours prior to doing your test, the presence of sugar in the urine will indicate only that the blood sugar has been high at some time during that period.

Clinitest

This test (Fig. 4.7a, page 70) requires the addition of urine to a tablet in a test tube and observing the colour change.

Equipment required

This includes:

- A test tube
- A dropper
- A container for urine
- Clinitest tablets.

Directions

1. Collect urine in a clean receptacle.

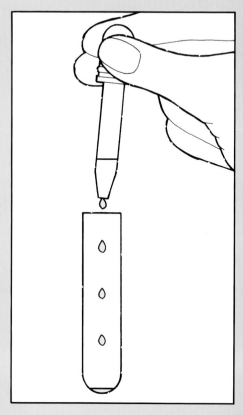

2. Draw urine into the dropper and place 5 drops into the test tube.

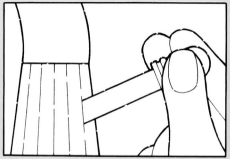

3. Rinse the dropper.

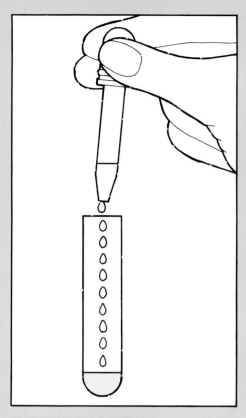

4. Draw water into the dropper and add 10 drops to the test tube.

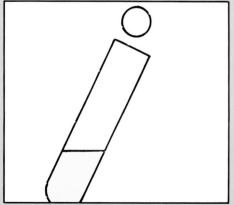

5. Drop one tablet into the test tube. Watch while the complete bubbling reaction takes place (see Interpretation of results page 192). <u>Do not shake</u> the tube during the reaction, nor for 15 seconds after the bubbling has stopped.

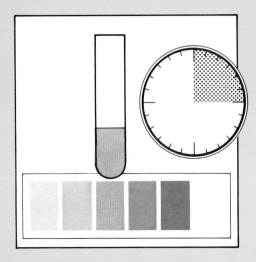

6. After the 15 seconds waiting period, shake the test tube gently and compare the colour of the liquid with the colour chart provided and note down the per cent result.

Note: For accurate results, always use special Clinitest droppers and test tubes, which can be obtained from your pharmacy.

Interpretation of the results

NEGATIVE — no sugar (glucose)

The liquid will be blue at the end of the waiting period of 15 seconds. The whitish sediment that may form has no bearing on the test and should be ignored.

POSITIVE — sugar present

The more sugar in the urine, the greater the colour change and the more rapidly it occurs. The amount of sugar is determined by comparing the colour of the solution in the test tube with the colour chart, at the end of the 15 second waiting period. Colour changes developing after the 15 second waiting period should be disregarded.

IMPORTANT

It is essential that you carefully observe the solution in the test tube while the bubbling reaction takes place and during the 15 second waiting period, in order to detect the rapid 'pass-through' colour changes. If the colours rapidly pass through green, tan and orange to a dark greenish-brown, you should record the result as over 2% sugar, without comparing the final colour development with the colour chart.

The colour chart and the above instructions must be used with Clinitest Reagent Tablets only.

Care and handling of Clinitest Reagent Tablets

- Keep tablets away from direct heat and sunlight (but not in a refrigerator).

- Replace bottle cap <u>immediately</u> after removing the tablet and before starting the test, since the tablets absorb moisture and spoil (turning dark blue) if the bottle is not kept tightly closed.

- Handle tablets cautiously; they contain caustic soda.

Diastix

Diastix (Fig. 4.7b, page 70) involves placing a strip of special paper in the stream of urine and then observing the colour change.

Equipment required

This test requires Diastix strips only.

Directions

1. Remove test strip from the bottle and replace the cap promptly and tightly.

    It is important that you:
    - <u>Do not touch</u> the test area of the strip.
    - <u>Use only the reagent strips with the pale blue test areas</u> (similar in colour to the 'negative' colour block of the colour chart on the bottle label).
    - Do not remove the small packet of moisture – absorbing crystals from the bottle.

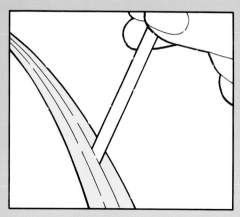

2. Dip the reagent strip into the stream of urine for 2 seconds and remove.

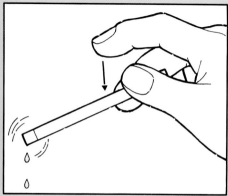

3. Tap the edge of the strip to remove excess urine.

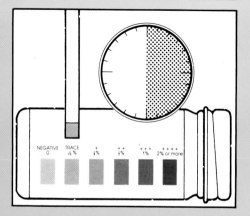

4. Wait 30 seconds and then immediately compare the colour of the test area against the Diastix colour chart, which ranges from 0% (blue) to 2% or more (brown). Record the result.

Note If you are using Keto-Diastix ignore the strips with the buff coloured test area, which are used for the measurement of ketones.

Diabur-Test 5000

The procedure with Diabur-Test 5000 (Fig. 4.7c, page 70) is similar to that for Diastix.

Equipment required

Diabur-Test 5000 test strips.

Directions

1. Remove a strip from the container.

2. Briefly dip the strip into the stream of urine or specimen.

3. Shake off the excess urine.

4. Wait 2 minutes.

5. Compare the colour of the test area with the Diabur colour scale and record the result.

TESTING FOR KETONES

Ketostix and Keto-Diastix

Equipment required

Keto-Diastix Ketostix or test strips.

Directions

The procedure is similar to that for Diastix and Diabur-Test 5000.

1. Remove a strip from the container.

2. Dip the strip into the stream of urine for a second or two.

3. Tap the edge of the strip to remove excess urine.

4. Wait <u>15 seconds.</u>

5. Compare the ketone test area with the ketone colour chart.

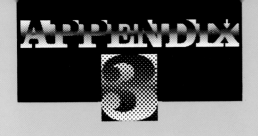
BLOOD TESTS

All blood tests (see page 64) depend on obtaining a small drop of blood, which is most readily obtained by pricking a finger, and putting it onto a specially prepared strip. The blood sugar level is determined by comparing the change in colour of the strip with the colour chart supplied with the test kit. Alternatively, the change in colour of the test strip is measured with a meter.

Procedure for blood tests

Equipment required

This includes:
- Test strips
- Finger pricker
- A paper tissue
- Strip reading meter — optional
- A wash bottle — only necessary with Dextrostix.

Obtaining the blood

Blood can be obtained from any part of the body, using the finger pricker (Fig. 4.1, page 64) — people prefer the finger or thumb, some the lobe of the ear!

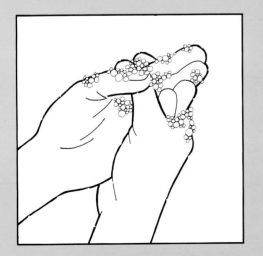

1. Wash your hands (or ear!) in warm water, then dry them.

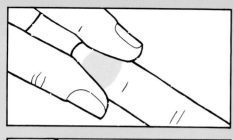

2. Squeeze the area to be pricked until it goes pink.

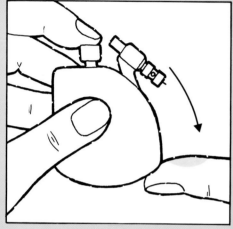

3. Prick firmly, using needle provided (or automatic pricker).

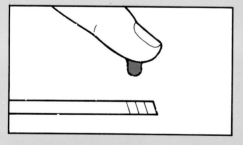

4. Make sure you have a good-sized drop of blood.

5. Allow the drop to fall onto the strip — do not smear or press it on.

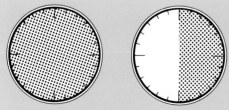

6. Start timing: 60 seconds with BM-Test Glycemie 20-800, or 30 seconds with Visidex II (with some machines timing is automatic).

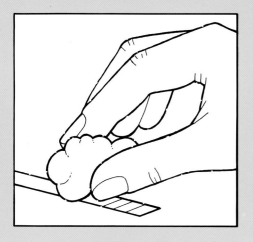

7. At the end of the time period, wash or wipe the blood off the strip.

The exact method depends on the type of strip you use. If washing, this must be performed carefully with the fine-jet bottle provided, or faulty results will be obtained.

Determining the blood sugar level

Visual colour comparison

Using the BM-Test Glycemie 20-800 or Visidex II, the colour change of the strip is visually compared with the colour chart provided (Fig. A3.1), in order to determine the blood sugar level.

Fig. A3.1.
Visual determination of the blood sugar level.

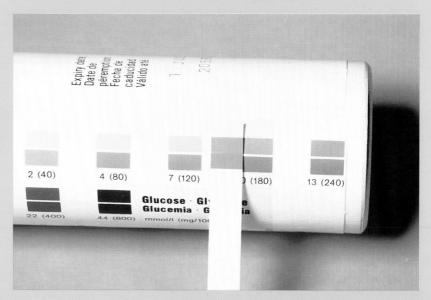

Measuring the colour change using a meter

In this type of blood test, the change in colour is measured with a meter (Fig. A3.2).

As the exact procedures vary with each meter, instructions are not given here. Whichever meter you use, the testing procedure must be followed carefully if you are to obtain accurate results.

Fig. A3.2.
Determining the blood sugar level using a meter.

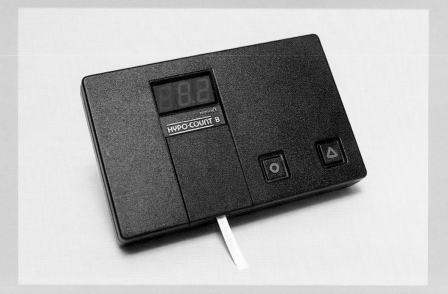

IMPORTANT

Various meters are available and it is absolutely essential that the correct strip is used with each meter. Before buying a meter, check with your doctor whether it is necessary.

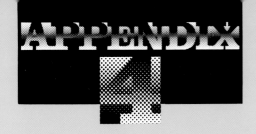

TREATING SEVERE HYPOGLYCAEMIA WITH GLUCAGON

ERRATUM: Since publication the glucagon pack has been changed. Please study the instructions which come with the pack.

Glucagon has the opposite effect to insulin. If you have a severe reaction, particularly if it results in unconsciousness, glucagon may be injected under the skin.

When consciousness is regained, carbohydrate, such as milk, must be given to prevent the reaction recurring.

How to administer glucagon

Equipment required

Glucagon is supplied in a kit form containing:

- A needle in a protective case (the case also serves as the syringe plunger)
- A syringe containing sterile water
- A vial containing glucagon powder.

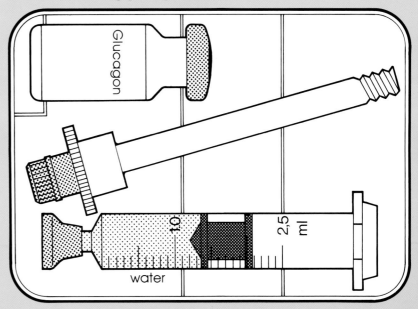

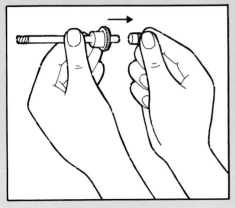

Procedure for assembling the syringe and drawing up the dose

It is worthwhile practising the assembly of the syringe and drawing up the glucagon before the occurrence of a severe reaction, when you may be flustered.

1. Remove the grey cap from the needle case (plunger).

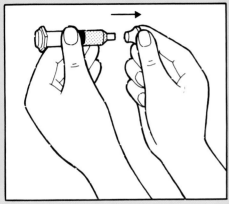

2. Remove the grey rubber cap from the syringe.

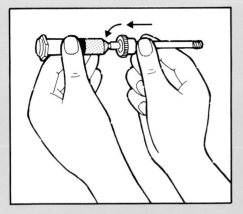

3. Leaving the needle inside the plunger, attach the needle to the syringe, pushing and twisting it gently.

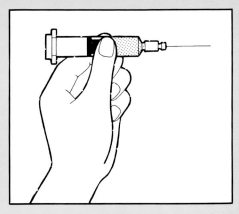

4. Remove the plunger, thereby exposing the needle.

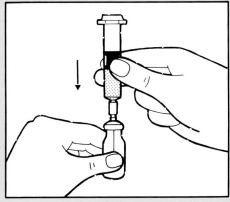

5. Pierce the blue rubber disk of the glucagon vial cap with the needle.

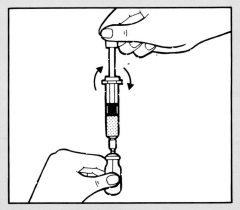

6. Screw the plunger into the syringe by inserting it through the green cap on the syringe and twisting it until it is tight.

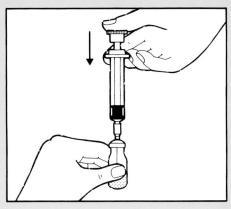

7. Add the water in the syringe to the glucagon in the vial by depressing the plunger.

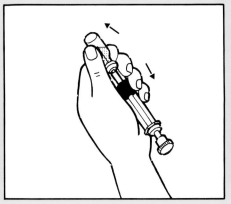

8. With the needle still inserted in the vial, turn the vial upside down and shake the contents until the tablet is dissolved — the fluid will be cloudy.

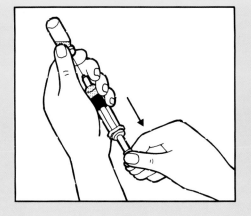

9. Withdraw the needle slightly, so that it is just piercing the blue rubber disk of the vial cap. Draw up the fluid into the syringe.

Giving the injection of glucagon

It is best to give glucagon as an intramuscular injection, which is why the needle supplied is longer than the needle usually used to inject insulin. The injection may be given in:

- The upper arm
- The thigh
- The top, outer quarter of the buttock.

No harm will be done if the injection accidentally goes into a blood vessel.

To give the injection proceed as follows:

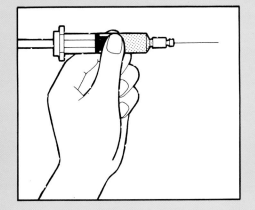

1. Hold the barrel of the syringe in either hand.

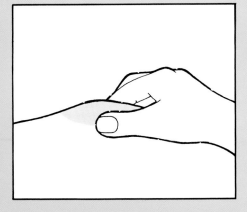

2. Pinch up a lump of muscle in your other hand.

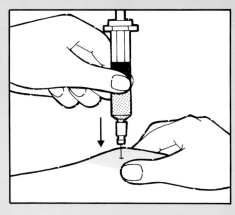

3. Still holding the barrel of the syringe, push the needle into the muscle for about three-quarters of its length.

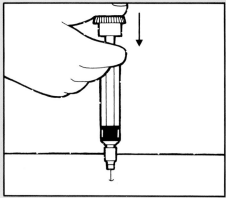

4. Depress the plunger until the whole dose has been given.

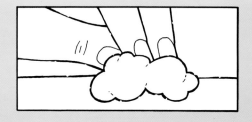

5. Withdraw the needle and hold a piece of cotton wool over the site for a few seconds.

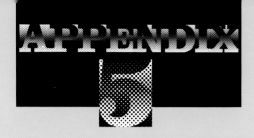

FOOD VALUES FOR THOSE WITH DIABETES

The first column in the following tables, with the exception of Tables II and VII, lists foods that provide 10 grams of carbohydrate when eaten in the amount stated. The amount is described in either of two ways:

1. A weight measured in grams (g)
2. A spoon measure.

If using the spoon measures, use standard kitchen measuring spoons, as used in compiling this list. The tablespoon (tbsp) measurement is based on a 15ml spoon, the teaspoon (tsp) on a 5ml spoon (all are level spoonsful).

Each item of food, if eaten in the amount stated (either the gram weight or spoon measure), will provide 10 grams of carbohydrate, i.e. 1 'exchange', 1 'portion' or 1 'line'.

For the overweight, the energy (calorie) intake is most important, and therefore the calorie content of each serving of food is given in the third column.

It is generally recommended that at least half of your carbohydrate allowance should come from the foods listed in the tables for starch (Table I) and vegetables (TABLES V and X). Also, the foods marked with an asterisk are all good (*) or very good (* *) sources of fibre, and it is recommended that you include as many of these as possible in your diet each day.

WEIGHTS AND MEASURES

Most diet scales are marked in metric weights, i.e. grams, and we recommend that you use this scale if weighing. If you only have scales marked in imperial weights, i.e. pounds and ounces, the following conversion charts may be useful:

Grams (g)		Approx. ounces
25	=	1
50	=	2
75	=	3
100	=	4
150	=	5
175	=	6
200	=	7

Millilitres (ml)		Approx. pints
75	=	$\frac{1}{8}$
150	=	$\frac{1}{4}$
275	=	$\frac{1}{2}$
425	=	$\frac{3}{4}$
550	=	1

TABLE I	Starchy foods
TABLE II	Bread
TABLE III	Breakfast cereals
TABLE IV	Biscuits, crackers, crispbreads
TABLE V	Vegetables
TABLE VI	Fruits
TABLE VII	Vegetables and some fruits
TABLE VIII	Fruit juices
TABLE IX	Processed foods
TABLE X	Milk and milk products
TABLE XI	Low-carbohydrate, high-calorie foods
TABLE XII	Alcoholic drinks

TABLE I

STARCHY FOODS	Approximate measure	Approximate weight of food (g) containing 10g carbohydrate	Calorie content
Arrowroot/custard powder/cornflour	1 tbsp	10	35
Barley, raw	1 tbsp	10	40
Flour, plain, white	1½ tbsp	10	40
Flour, self-raising, white	1½ tbsp	10	45
* Flour, wholemeal, wholewheat	2 tbsp	15	50
**Oats, uncooked	3 tbsp	15	60
Spaghetti, white, uncooked	6 long (19") strands	10	45
**Spaghetti, wholewheat, uncooked	20 short (10") strands	15	50
* Spaghetti/macaroni, cooked	2 tbsp	10	45
Rice, white, uncooked	1 tbsp	10	45
**Rice, brown, uncooked	1 tbsp	10	40
Sago/tapioca/semolina, uncooked	2 tsp	10	35
* Soya flour, full fat	14 tbsp	75	300
* Soya flour, low fat	9 tbsp	50	125
* Soya granules, dry	13 tbsp	75	200

* Good fibre content
**Very good fibre content

TABLE II

BREAD	Size of loaf	Type of bread	Approximate weight of carbohydrate (g)	Calorie content
1 thin slice	small	wholemeal*	10	50
1 thin slice	small	white	10	50
1 thin slice	large	wholemeal*	13	69
1 thin slice	large	white	15	75
1 thick slice	large	wholemeal*	20	100
1 thick slice	large	white	26	125
1 roll		wholemeal*	13	69
1 roll		white	15	75

*Good fibre content

TABLE III

BREAKFAST CEREALS	Approximate measure	Approximate weight of food (g) containing 10g carbohydrate	Calorie content
**Allbran	5 tbsp	20	50
**Bran Buds	4 tbsp	20	50
Cornflakes	5 tbsp	10	40
**Muesli (unsweetened)	2 tbsp	15	50
**Muesli (sweetened)	2 tbsp	15	55
**Puffed Wheat	15 tbsp	15	50
Rice Krispies	6 tbsp	10	40
**Shredded Wheat	2/3 of one		80
Special K	8 tbsp	15	50
**Spoonsize Cubs	12-14		45
**Weetabix	1		60
**Weetaflakes	4 tbsp	15	50

**Very good fibre content

Values for all individual breakfast cereals are given in 'Countdown'.

TABLE IV

BISCUITS, CRACKERS, CRISPBREADS	Approximate measure	Approximate weight of food (g) containing 10g carbohydrate	Calorie content
Biscuits, plain	2	15	60
**Biscuits, digestive or wholemeal	1	15	70
Biscuits, cream or chocolate	1	10	60
Crackers, plain	2	15	70
Crispbread	2	15	50

**Good fibre content

Values for individual biscuits are given in 'Countdown'.

TABLE V

VEGETABLES+	Approximate measure	Approximate weight of food (g) containing 10g carbohydrate	Calorie content
**Beans, baked	4 tbsp	75	55
**Beans, broad, boiled	10 tbsp	150	75
**Beans, dried, all types, raw	2 tbsp	20	55
*Beetroot, cooked, whole	2 small	100	45
*Lentils, dry, raw	2 tbsp	20	60
*Onions, raw	1 large	200	45
*Parsnips, raw	1 small	90	45
*Peas, marrow fat or processed	7 tbsp	75	60
*Peas, dried, all types, raw	2 tbsp	20	60
*Plantain, green, raw, peeled	small slice	35	40
*Potatoes, raw	1 small egg-sized	50	45
*Potatoes, boiled	1 small egg-sized	50	40
*Potatoes, chips (weighed when cooked)	4-5 chips	25	65
**Potatoes, jacket (weighed with skin)	1 small-sized	50	45
*Potatoes, mashed	1 small scoop	50	80
*Potatoes, roast	½ medium-sized	40	65
*Sweetcorn, canned or frozen	5 tbsp	60	45
**Sweetcorn, on the cob	½ medium cob	75	60
*Sweet potato, raw, peeled	1 small slice	50	45

* Good fibre content
** Very good fibre content
+ Vegetables which can be eaten freely are listed in TABLE X

TABLE VI

FRUITS+	Approximate measure	Approximate weight of food (g) containing 10g carbohydrate	Calorie content
*Apples, eating, whole	1 medium	110	50
*Apples, cooking, whole	1 medium	125	55
*Apples, stewed without sugar	6 tbsp	125	40
*Apricots, fresh, whole	3 medium	160	40
*Apricots, dried, raw	4 small	25	45
*Bananas, whole	5½" in length	90	40
*Bananas, peeled	3½" in length	50	40
*Bilberries, raw	5 tbsp	75	40
*Blackberries, raw	10 tbsp	150	45
*Blackcurrants, raw	10 tbsp	150	45
*Cherries, fresh, whole	12	100	40
*Currants, dried	2 tbsp	15	35
*Damsons, raw, whole	7	120	40
*Dates, fresh, whole	3 medium	50	40
*Dates, dried, without stones	3 small	15	40
*Figs, fresh, whole	1	100	40
*Figs, dried	1	20	45
*Grapes, whole	10 large	75	40
*Grapefruit, whole	1 very large	400	45
*Greengages, fresh, whole	5	90	40
*Guavas, fresh, peeled	1	70	45
*Mango, fresh, whole	⅓ of a large one	100	40

FRUITS+	Approximate measure	Approximate weight of food (g) containing 10g carbohydrate	Calorie content
Melon, all types, weighed with skin	large slice	300	40
*Nectarine, fresh, whole	1	90	40
*Orange, fresh, whole	1 large	150	40
*Pawpaw, fresh, whole	$\frac{1}{6}$ of a large one	80	50
*Peach, fresh, whole	1 large	125	40
*Pears, fresh, whole	1 large	130	40
*Pineapple, fresh, no skin or core	1 thick slice	90	40
*Plums, cooking, fresh, whole	4 medium	180	40
*Plums, dessert, fresh, whole	2 large	110	40
*Pomegranate, fresh, whole	1 small	110	40
*Prunes, dried, without stones	2 large	25	40
*Raisins, dried	2 tbsp	15	35
*Raspberries, fresh	12 tbsp	175	45
*Strawberries, fresh	15 medium	160	40
*Sultanas, dried	2 tbsp	15	40
*Tangerines, fresh, whole	2 large	175	40

* Good fibre content

+ A few fruits contain very little natural sugar and can be taken in generous helpings without counting calories, e.g. cranberries, gooseberries, lemons, loganberries and rhubarb — all other fruits should be counted into your diet.

TABLE VII

VEGETABLES AND SOME FRUITS

The following foods contain no more than 5g of carbohydrate and 20—25 calories in a normal (approximately 100g/ 4oz) serving:

VEGETABLES

*Artichokes, cooked	*Lettuce
*Asparagus, cooked	*Marrow, cooked
*Aubergine, cooked	*Mushrooms, raw
*Beans, fresh runner	Mustard and cress
*Beansprouts, raw	Okra, raw
*Broccoli	*Onions, boiled
**Brussels sprouts	Peppers
**Cabbage, raw	*Pumpkin
**Carrots, cooked	Radishes
*Cauliflower, cooked	Spinach, boiled
**Celery, raw or cooked	*Swede, boiled
*Courgettes	*Tomatoes, raw and canned
*Cucumber	*Turnip
**Leeks, cooked	Watercress

REMEMBER: White sauces count!

FRUITS

Cranberries	Loganberries	Melon
*Currants, red and black	Grapefruit (½)	*Raspberries
Gooseberries	Lemons	Rhubarb

*Good fibre content
**Very good fibre content

TABLE VIII

FRUIT JUICES+	Approximate measure	Approximate weight of food (g) containing 10g carbohydrate	Calorie content
Apple juice, unsweetened	6 tbsp	85	40
Blackcurrant, unsweetened	7 tbsp	100	40
Grapefruit, unsweetened	8 tbsp	125	45
Orange, unsweetened	7 tbsp	100	40
Pineapple, unsweetened	6 tbsp	85	40
Tomato, unsweetened	1 large glass	275	50

+The carbohydrate value will vary slightly according to the time of year.

TABLE IX

PROCESSED FOODS+	Approximate measure	Approximate weight of food (g) containing 10g carbohydrate	Calorie content
FOODS			
Beefburgers, frozen	3 small	—	450
Canned soup	½ medium tin (thick)	—	170
Fish fingers	2	—	110
Complan	3 tbsp	—	
Ice-cream	1 scoop	—	90
Sausages	2 thick	110	400
Scotch egg	½	—	180
DRINKS			
Beer, draught	½ pint		100
Lager, draught	¾ pint		135
Cider, dry	¾ pint		120
Cider, sweet	½ pint		95
Cider, vintage	¼ pint		75

+ This table lists a few typical foods and drinks which provide approximately 10g of carbohydrate. As there are considerable variations between the products marketed by different manufacturers, it is recommended that if your family uses processed foods regularly, you should refer to the comprehensive lists of manufactured foods and alcoholic drinks provided in 'Countdown'.

TABLE X

MILK AND MILK PRODUCTS	Approximate measure	Approximate weight of food (g) containing 10g carbohydrate	Calorie content
Milk, fresh	1 cup	200	130
Milk, fresh, semi-skimmed	1 cup	200	95
Milk, fresh, skimmed	1 cup	200	70
Milk, dried, whole	8 tsps	25	125
Milk, dried, skimmed	10 tsps	20	70
Milk, evaporated	6 tblsp	90	145
Yoghurt, plain, low fat	1 small carton	150	80

TABLE XI

LOW-CARBOHYDRATE, HIGH-CALORIE FOODS +	Approximate measure	Approximate weight of food (g)	Calorie content
DAIRY PRODUCTS			
Butter/margarine	5 tsp	25	185
Low fat spreads	5 tsp	25	95
Egg — medium uncooked	1	55	80
Cream, single	Small pot	150	320
Cream, double	Small pot	150	670
Cream, whipped	Small pot	150	500
Cheese, Cheddar	Small matchbox size	25	100
Cheese, cottage	5 tbsp	100	110
Cheese, cream	1 heaped tbsp	25	110
Cheese, Edam	Small matchbox size	25	75
Cheese, Parmesan	3 tbsp	25	100
Cheese, Quark	Small pot	100	90
Cheese, Stilton	Small matchbox size	25	115
Cheese spread	3 tbsp	50	140
MEAT			
Bacon, lean, grilled	1 rasher	25	75
Bacon, lean, fried	1 rasher	25	80
Bacon, streaky, grilled	1 rasher	25	105
Bacon, streaky, fried	1 rasher	25	125
Meat, lean, raw	1 av. helping	100	125
Meat, lean, cooked	1 av. helping	100	160
Meat, fatty, raw	1 av. helping	100	410
Poultry, white meat, cooked	1 av. helping	100	140
Poultry, dark meat, cooked	1 av. helping	100	155
Lamb, cutlet, grilled	1 medium	100	250
Pork chop, grilled	1 medium	150	390
Corned beef	2 slices	50	110

LOW-CARBOHYDRATE, HIGH-CALORIE FOODS	Approximate measure	Approximate weight of food (g)	Calorie content
FISH			
Fish fillets, white, raw	1 av. helping	100	80
Fish fillets, oily, raw	1 av. helping	100	230
Shellfish, shelled	1 av. helping	100	80-100
NUTS			
Almonds, shelled	4 tbsp	50	280
Brazil, shelled	14 medium	50	310
Hazelnuts, shelled	6 tbsp	50	190
Coconut, dried	5 tbsp	25	150
Peanuts, roast	1 small packet	25	145
Walnuts	16 halves	50	130
MISCELLANEOUS			
Oil, vegetable	1 tbsp	15	135
Suet, shredded	6 tbsp	50	420

+NOTE: Because the foods and drinks listed in TABLE XI contain a high calorie content, particular care is required if you are overweight.

TABLE XII

The carbohydrate and/or calorie content of a range of alcoholic drinks is listed below. If you are on insulin or large doses of oral hypoglycaemic agents you are reminded **NOT** to exchange alcohol for 'food exchanges' (portions). Providing you do not exceed recommended amount of 3 drinks a day (see page 54) the carbohydrate contribution can be ignored. We do not advise you to drink beers or lager/ciders that exceed an alcohol content of 5%.

Alcoholic drinks		Approximate measure	Carbohydrate (g)	Calorie content
Beer		per ½ pint	10	100/130
Cider, dry		per ½ pint	5	100
sweet		per ½ pint	10	100/120
Lager		per ½ pint	7-10	85/110
Vermouth, dry		1 pub measure (⅓ gill)	1-5	50/60
sweet		1 pub measure (⅓ gill)	5-10	70/80
Sherry, dry		1 pub measure (⅓ gill)	1-2	50/60
sweet		1 pub measure (⅓ gill)	5-10	70/90
Sparkling wine/Champagne	dry	4 fl oz/113ml glass	1-2	80/90
	sweet	4 fl oz/113ml glass	5-10	90/100
Wine (red/white) dry		4 fl oz/113ml glass	1-2	70/80
sweet		4 fl oz/113ml glass	5-10	80/100
Spirits, i.e. whisky, gin, rum, vodka, brandy, advocaat		1 pub measure ($\frac{1}{6}$ gill)	neg	50/70
Liqueurs		1 pub measure ($\frac{1}{6}$ gill)	5-10	80/100

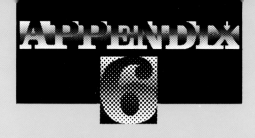

APPENDIX 8

INSULIN INFUSION PUMPS

Construction and function

The pumps, which are worn either on a belt or shoulder holster (Fig. 3.9, page 32) provide a small, continuous flow of insulin throughout the day and, by means of a mechanism controlled by the wearer, spurt insulin just before each meal.

Several pumps are available, varying in cost and level of sophistication. They are battery driven, and contain a reservoir or syringe which has to be replaced every 36-48 hours. Thin tubing connects the pump to a fine needle, which is inserted under the skin of the abdomen. The insulin flow rate can be varied, either by increasing the amount of insulin in the reservoir, or, as in the more sophisticated pumps, by means of an integral control panel. The peaks of insulin required before meals are supplied by setting the required amount on a dial or push-button control panel. In the most advanced — and most expensive — pumps, the continuous flow of insulin (basal rate) and the peak levels can be varied according to special programmes. Depending on the model, audible or visual signals are given should the pump stop or become disconnected.

Availability and use

Insulin infusion pumps are at present used only for those whose diabetes is difficult or impossible to control with traditional methods.

The procedures involved in using an infusion pump are complicated and vary according to the model. Individual instruction is always required and is beyond the scope of this Handbook.

Advantages

- They allow greater flexibility of meal times and the amounts of carbohydrate which can be eaten.
- For some people with diabetes they provide better overall control.

Disadvantages

- They are quite large and cumbersome, and some regard them as unsightly.
- They require close attention to ensure malfunction has not occured.
- Blood tests may be needed just as frequently as with traditional methods.
- Pump failures with existing models are still frequent.
- They have to be removed for sports, washing, sexual intercourse etc., and the needle resited afterwards.

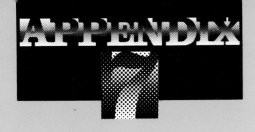
THE CHILD WITH DIABETES AT SCHOOL — GUIDELINES FOR TEACHERS

Diabetes — cause and symptoms

Diabetes results from a lack of insulin, which causes a rise in the blood sugar level. The child becomes ill, developing the typical symptoms, thirst and dehydration, passing large amounts of urine, and losing a considerable amount of weight.

Treatment of diabetes

Insulin

Children with diabetes need life-long treatment with insulin injections, given once or twice daily.

Diet

Insulin treatment must be balanced by a regular diet of known carbohydrate content. The child (or parents) will have a diet sheet and this, together with the help of the school meals service, will ensure that the child is provided with the right type of food.

Sugar and sugar-containing foods should be avoided, except in emergencies noted below. Protein foods (meat and fish) and most vegetables can be eaten freely. The carbohydrate (starch) intake needs to be fixed for each meal, and with the aid of the diet sheet this is simple to calculate. A small amount of carbohydrate is needed at 'elevenses' and teatime, in addition to the larger amounts taken at the main meals.

A child with diabetes can lead a normal school life and will be able to undertake all the activities enjoyed by other children, including sports, although extra food (such as sweets, sugar or biscuits) will be needed before the more vigorous activities, especially swimming.

Insulin reactions (hypoglycaemia)

Hypoglycaemia occurs either because too much insulin has been taken, or because insufficient carbohydrate has been eaten, for example, if meals are eaten very late or after vigorous physical exercise. Some of the following symptoms may occur:

- Lack of concentration, listlessness
- Pallor, sweating
- Stubbornness, difficulty in reading or answering questions
- Unreasonable tearfulness.

The child may also experience hunger, shakiness, numbness and tingling of the lips and tongue, double vision or headache, and vomiting. In the more advanced stages, the child may become unconscious, in which case medical help should be sought. These episodes are not dangerous.

Treatment of insulin reactions

If child or teacher notices the symptoms of an insulin reaction, sugar should be given at once: 2 heaped teaspoonsful or 3 lumps in water; or the child should suck Dextrosol (glucose) tablets, or sweets. Recovery normally occurs after a few minutes, at which time the child should be given an additional biscuit, chocolate or sandwich.

Prevention of insulin reactions

Every effort should be made to prevent reactions by making sure that they do not miss 'elevenses', that they are not too late for the mid-day meal, and above all that they take extra carbohydrate before strenuous exercise.

General hints

- **Inoculations** — children with diabetes may have the same inoculations and vaccinations as those without.

- **Dental treatment** — no special arrangements are needed, and there are no problems associated with local anaesthetics. If a general anaesthetic is needed, the hospital diabetic clinic should be consulted.

If you would like copies of Appendix 7, it is available in leaflet form, on request to: The British Diabetic Association,
10 Queen Anne Street,
London W1M 0BD.

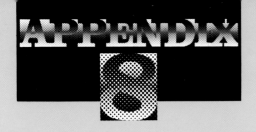

WHAT THE BABYSITTER NEEDS TO KNOW

Appendix 8 is based on a leaflet published by the B.D.A. which parents of children with diabetes can complete and leave with a babysitter. Copies are available on request to:

The British Diabetic Association,
10 Queen Anne Street,
London W1M 0BD.

To the Babysitter

_____ has diabetes

Diabetes means that my child's pancreas does not make enough insulin. Without insulin, food cannot be used properly. A child with diabetes must take daily injections of insulin and must balance his/her food and exercise.

An insulin reaction may occur if the blood sugar gets too low — especially before meals or after exercise.

WARNING SIGNS OF INSULIN REACTIONS

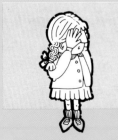
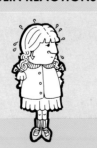
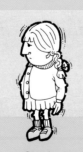
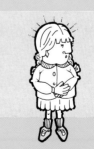
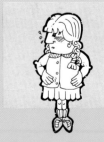

| Blurred vision | Perspiring, Paleness | Shaky, Nervous | Headache, Nausea, Stomach ache | Changes of mood, Confusion, Irritability, Tearfulness |

My child usually behaves as follows when having a reaction:

_____

_____

If this happens, give my child any of the following <u>immediately:</u>
   3 glucose tablets (e.g. Dextrosol)

<u>or</u> 2 teaspoons of sugar/glucose powder in water.

<u>or</u> 1 small cup (approx. 4 fl. oz./100ml) unsweetened fruit juice.

<u>or</u> between ⅓-½ of a 330ml can of sweetened fizzy drinks (e.g. Coke, lemonade, etc.)

<u>or</u> _____

You will find this supply of sugary foods and drinks

_____

Normally, you should follow this with a cup of milk and 2 biscuits or crackers

<u>or</u> _____

If my child does not improve in 10-15 minutes give him/her one of the above list again.

If my child still does not improve, call us/the emergency number/doctor.

A child with diabetes checks his/her urine/blood during the day to find out about his/her sugar level. There are various methods to use. We will show you the method we use.

NOTES FOR TODAY:

Test urine/blood at:

_____ _____ _____

and record below:

_____ _____ _____

Snacks or meals:

Serve _____

_____ at _____ o'clock

Serve _____

_____ at _____ o'clock

Serve _____

_____ at _____ o'clock

Parents are at:

_____ Phone _____

Emergency number is:

_____ Phone _____

Clinic consultant:

_____ Phone _____

NOTES:

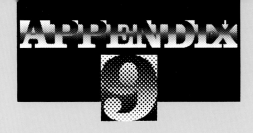

APPENDIX 9

B.D.A. PUBLICATIONS

Children's books

I HAVE DIABETES

A booklet in the popular Althea series for children and parents which explains diabetes as a story.
Colour illustrations

Diet and recipe books

BETTER COOKERY FOR DIABETICS

by BDA dietitian, Jill Metcalfe. Over 130 delicious and healthy recipes with practical hints for following the low fat, high fibre diet recommended for diabetics. Spiral bound, 16 pages of colour illustrations.

COOKING THE NEW DIABETIC WAY — THE HIGH FIBRE, CALORIE-CONSCIOUS COOKBOOK

compiled by BDA dietitian Jill Metcalfe. Over 260 low fat, reduced calories, high fibre recipes. A useful book for diabetics who need to lose weight. Recipes feature servings for two and four. Eight pages of colour illustrations.

VEGETARIAN ON A DIET

the high fibre, low sugar, low fat, wholefood vegetarian cook book by Margaret Cousins and Jill Metcalfe. An introduction to the benefits of the vegetarian way of eating with specific advice for the diabetic and weight watcher. Featuring a wide range of exciting but practical recipes with an extensive wholefood food values list. All recipes have complete carbohydrate and calorie counts.

COUNTDOWN

A guide to the carbohydrate and calorie content of manufactured foods and drinks.
Designed to help you choose your food wisely.

SIMPLE DIABETIC COOKERY

A booklet of 50 one and two serving high fibre recipes.

SIMPLE HOME BAKING

A booklet of 50 high fibre, reduced fat home baking recipes including cakes, biscuits and breads. The recipes range from basic bread to celebration cakes and all are carbohydrate and calorie calculated.

GLOSSARY

Acidosis
A build-up of acids, usually ketones, in the blood.

Acetone
Is a sweet smelling ketone that may be smelt on the breath of people with ketones in the blood.

Adrenalin
Is the hormone released from the central portion of the adrenal glands in response to a stress or emergency, e.g. an illness, a hypoglycaemic reaction, a fright.

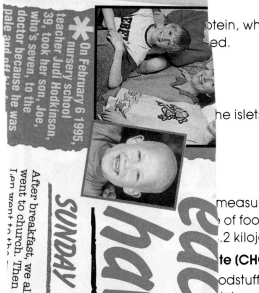

...tein, which may appear in the urine when the kidneys ...ed.

...he islets of Langerhans in the pancreas that produce

...measurement of heat or energy used to assess the ... of food. It is being replaced by the kilojoule. ...2 kilojoules.

...te (CHO)
...odstuff that is an important source of energy to the ...inly represented by sugars and starches.

Cataract
An opacity in the lens of the eye that may be caused by long-standing diabetes.

Coma
A state of unconsciousness. In diabetes this can result from severe hypoglycaemia or severe keto-acidosis.

Cortisol
A hormone released from the outer portion of the adrenal glands during stress, shock, infection, etc.

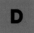

Dehydration
Refers to being depleted of water. It occurs when the blood sugar is high for long periods, as in keto-acidosis.

Dextrose
Simply sugar (see glucose).

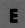

Electrolytes
A term applied to the important salts of the body, such as sodium, potassium, chlorides and bicarbonate.

Enuresis
Involuntary passage of urine, bedwetting.

Exchange diet
One in which a fixed number of servings of carbohydrate, fat, protein and milk foods is prescribed so as to control total energy intake as well as the quantities of all major foodstuffs.

Fat atrophy
Disappearance of fat from under the skin, at the site of insulin injection. More common with less refined insulins.

Fat hypertrophy
Swelling of the fat where insulin is being injected.

Fatty acids
These are the main components of body fat in which they are combined with glycerol (glycerine).

Fructose

A sugar occurring in fruit, a simple carbohydrate.

Gangrene

Death of tissue due to poor blood supply.

Glucose

Simple sugar.

Glucagon

A hormone produced by cells of the islets of Langerhans in the pancreas. It tends to raise the blood sugar level.

Gluconeogenesis

The making of glucose by the liver, especially from protein breakdown products.

Glycogen

Is made by the body from glucose and is the main complex CHO in animals. It is stored in the liver and muscles.

Glycogenolysis

The process of releasing glucose from glycogen stored in the liver.

Glycosuria

The presence of sugar in the urine.

Haemoglobin A, (glycosylated haemoglobin)

A test used to assess long-term diabetic control.

Hormone

The name given to a chemical substance released by an organ into the bloodstream. Hormones are responsible for controlling such functions as metabolism, growth, sex development, blood sugar levels, etc.

Hyperglycaemia

A high blood sugar.

Hypoglycaemia or 'hypo'

A low blood sugar (less than 3 mmol/l).

Insulin

A hormone produced by the beta cells in the islets of Langerhans in the pancreas. It enables glucose in the blood to get into the cells and be used for energy or to be stored.

Insulin reaction

Another term for hypoglycaemic reaction.

Intestine

The gut or bowel between the stomach and the anus.

Intravenous glucose

This is glucose that is injected directly into a vein.

Intravenous infusion

Liquid, such as water containing salt and glucose, being slowly injected, usually out of a bottle and over a long period of time, directly into the bloodstream via a vein.

Keto-acidosis or ketosis

A state of overproduction of ketones in the body which causes a build-up of acids in the blood.

Ketones

When fats are broken down in the body, ketones are produced. If a lot of fat is broken down, as in poorly controlled diabetes, the ketones accumulate in the blood, pass into the urine and can be smelt on the breath.

Ketonuria

The presence of ketones in the urine.

L

Lactose
The sugar found in milk.

Lipolysis
Breakdown of fat caused by starvation or lack of insulin.

M

Metabolism
The system of chemical control in the body.

Ml
Millilitre, a measure of volume.

mmol/l
Millimole per litre, a measure of the concentration of a substance.

N

Neuropathy
A disorder of the nerves, where the signals in them are not properly conducted. It is sometimes seen in those with diabetes.

O

Ophthalmologist
An eye specialist.

P

Pancreas
A long organ lying across the back of the abdomen. Part of it secretes digestive juices into the intestine, but its islets of Langerhans, pinpoint sized collections of cells scattered throughout it like currants in a cake, secrete insulin and glucagon.

Polydipsia
Excessive thirst.

Polyuria
The passing of large quantities of urine, and in diabetes caused

when there is overflow into the urine of excess glucose from the bloodstream.

Portion

One portion equals 10 grams of carbohydrate in this book.

Portion diet

One in which only the carbohydrate-containing foods are carefully prescribed in quantity in terms of 'portions'.

Post-prandial

After the meal.

Protein

A major food component important in body building, but may provide energy.

Reaction

See hypoglycaemia

Renal threshold

The level of sugar in the blood above which it spills over into the urine.

Retina

The light-receptive layer at the back of the eye. It is an extension of the optic nerve in the eye.

Retinopathy

Damage to the retina. May be caused by long-standing diabetes.

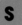

Sorbitol

A sweetening agent which when absorbed is converted in the liver to fructose.

Sucrose

Cane sugar.

Thrush

A fungal infection of nails, skin, mouth or vagina.

Triglyceride

A combination of fats used to carry or store fats in the body.

Unit

Refers to a quantity chosen as a standard basic measurement of insulin.

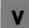

Vitamins

Compounds found in small quantities in natural foods. They are required for normal growth and maintenance of life, although they do not themselves provide energy or substance.

INDEX

A

Acidosis see Keto-acidosis
Accidents
    causing diabetes, 7
    insurance, 121
Adoption, 115
Air travel, 129-31
Alcohol, 54, 221
    driving and, 136
    exchange values, 218
Allergy to insulin, 185
Anxiety, see Stress
Appetite increase, 18
Arterial disease, 100-1
Autolet pricker, 64

B

Babies born to diabetic mothers, 113
Babysitters, guidelines for, 227-9
'Balance', 140
Beers, diabetic, 136
Beverages see Drinks
Biscuits, 40, 212
Blindness, insulin injection aids for, 186
Blood sugar meter, 66,200
Blood sugar
    balancing with insulin, 22
    effect of exercise on, 60
    effect of meals on, 31, 77

    effect of illness and stress on, 62
    effect of no insulin on, 16-17
    high blood sugar see Hyperglycaemia
    low blood sugar see Hypoglycaemia
    normal range, 67
    effect of food on, 4, 14-15
    source, 11
    storage of excess, 11
    testing see Blood tests
Blood tests, 197-200
    see also Tests for sugar
    aids for the blind, 106
    during keto-acidosis, 82
    equipment, 197
    essential, 68
    frequency, 68
    in children, 150
    interpretation, 67-68
    measuring colour change with
      meter, 200
    obtaining sample, 197-9
    pregnancy and, 111
    pregnancy after, 114
    technique, 64-66
Types of test
    BM-Test Glycemie 20-800, 65, 199
    Dextrostix, 197
    Visidex 11, 65, 199
    visual colour comparison, 199
BM-Test Glycemie 20-800, 65, 199
Bread, 47
    exchange values, 40, 210
Breakfast
    normal-sized, 86
    small, 86
Breast feeding, 114
British Diabetic Association, 139-41

C

Caesarian section, 112
Calluses, 98
Calories,
Camps for children, 160
Carbohydrate
  exchanges, 40-41, 207-22
  extra requirements for exercise, 93,
    123, 155
  foods containing, 34-35
  low-carbohydrate, high calories food
    and drinks, 220-1
  meal timing and, 37-38
  rapidly absorbed types, 47-48
  requirements, 38
Cataracts, 98
Causes of diabetes, 6-7
Cereals, 47
  exchange values, 40, 211
Childbirth, 112
Children
  adoption, 115
  at school, 154-9
  — guidelines for teachers, 225-6
  food problems in, 151-2
  holidays general, 159
  holidays, camps, 160
  hypoglycaemia in, 146-51
  ignoring diabetes, 163
  injecting themselves, 144-5
  injections in small children, 144-6
  insulin dose, adjustments in, 153-4
  leaving in care of others, 154, 159-60,
    227-9
  likelihood of diabetes development
    in, 109
  manipulating parents, 163-4
  reactions to diabetes in family, 167
  social activities, 164-5
  teaching about diabetes, 162-3
  test in, 152-3
  travel, 161-2
Clinics
  attendance at, 103
  organization, 101
Clinistix, 189
Clinitest, 70-71, 189-93
Coma, cause of, 18
  see also Keto-acidosis
Complications of diabetes, 20
  prevention, 21-22
Conferences on diabetes, 141
Contraception, 115-16
Convulsions in children, 147-9
Corns, 98
Crackers, 212
Crispbread, 212

D

Dairy products, 220
  high fat, 50
  low fat, 45
Dances, 132-3
Definition of diabetes, 3-4
Dehydration, 128
Dentistry, 104-5
  in children, 165
Diabetes (general only: see also Insulin
    dependent diabetes; Non- insulin
    dependent diabetes)
  causes, 6-8
  definition, 3-4
  history, 1-3
  how it develops, 4-5

long-term effects, 20
— prevention of, 21-22
research into, 141
statistics, 1, 6
symptoms, 9, 17
treatment, 10
types, 5
'Diabetic' beers, 136
foods, 53
Diabetic retinopathy, 99
Diabur-Test 5000, 70, 189, 195
Diastix, 70, 189, 193-5
Diet
see also Food; Meals; Snacks
for family, 57-58, 167-8
general principles, 42
guidelines for children at school, 225
planning, 37, 59
Dieting see Weight loss
Discos, 132-3
Drinks, 45, 46
alcohol, 54
during hypoglycaemia, 89
during keto-acidosis, 82
exchange values, 83, 217-19
low carbohydrate, high calorie, 220-1
Driving
alcohol and, 136
hypoglycaemia and, 136
insurance, 135
licence application, 134
prohibitions on, 135
Drugs
causing diabetes, 8
diabetes and, 137

E

Eating out, 55-56
Ebers Papyrus, 1, 2
Educating children about diabetes, 162-3
Emigration, 132
Employment, diabetes and, 117-20
Equipment
insulin injections, 169
urine tests, 189
blood tests, 197
Energy
production, 11-12
stores, breakdown of, 17, 19
Exchanges, carbohydrate, 40-41, 207-22
Exercise
at school, 155-8
causing hypoglycaemia, 92-93
diet adjustment for, 60, 155
effect on blood sugar, 15-16, 60
effect of unexpected, 87, 157-8
insulin dose adjustment for, 60
prohibited, 123-4, 157
Eye damage, 98-99
prevention, 99

F

Family planning, 114
Fats
breakdown of, 5
dietary, 36, 49-50
storage, 11
Fear of insulin injection, 184
Feet
corns and calluses, 98
damage to, 95
— prevention of damage, 95-98
first aid for, 98

heat and cold effects on, 97
inspection, 95-96
nail cutting, 97
shoes, 97-98
washing, 96
Fertility, 108
Fibre in foods, 36, 43, 44, 209-16
Finance, 120-1
Fish, 221
Fluids see Drinks
Food
see also Diet; Meals; Snacks
basic components, 33-36
carbohydrate content, 38-41
— exchanges, 83, 207-22
changing the amount, 77
'diabetic', 53
during hypoglycaemia, 89
effects on blood sugar, 4, 14,-15
extra food during exercise, 93, 155
low carbohydrate, high calorie, 220-1
problems in children, 151-2
sickness, during
timing of, p. 31
types, 42
to avoid, 51-52
to eat freely, 46
to eat in regulated amounts, 47-48
to eat regularly, 43-46
to eat with caution, 49-50
Football, 123-4
see also Exercise
Fruit, 43, 44, 46
exchange values, 41, 214-16
Fruit Juices, 217

G
Genital soreness, 17
Glucagon therapy during
hypoglycaemia, 91
for small children, 148
injection technique, 201-6
Glucose see Sugar
Glycogen storage in liver, 11
Glycosuria, 16-17

H
Heredity of diabetes, 6, 7, 8, 109, 167
History of diabetes, 1-3
Holidays
for adults, 125-31, 141,
for children, 140, 159-60
Hospitalization
diabetic controls, and during, 105
for childbirth, 112
Hyperglycaemia
causes, 16
effects, 17-20
Hypoglycaemia
causes, 15
driving and, 136
effect on intelligence, 150-1
glucagon treatment of, 201-6
guidelines for teachers, 225-6
in small children, 146-51
informing friends about, 91
occurring at school, 154-5, 157, 225-6
occurring at work, 118-19
precautions, 90
preventing, 92-94
recognizing, 150
symptoms, 88
treatment, 89
when it can occur, 85-87

I

Identity card, 126
Illness
   causing diabetes, 7-8
   effect on blood sugar, 62
   effect on diabetes, 104
   in children, 165-6
   insurance, 121, 129
   on holiday, 162
Immunization, 126
   for children, 162
Impotence, 100
Infection
   at injection site, 185
   from high blood sugar, and, 20
Infusion pumps, 31.223-4
Injections see Insulin
Injector guns, 146, 184
Insulin
   allergy to, 185
   availability abroad, 127
   balancing with blood sugar, 22
   clear (quick-acting), 23-24
   — effects of varying doses of, 26-29
   — injection timing for travellers, 131
   — maximum effect of, 94
   cloudy (slow-acting), 23-25
   — effects of varying doses of, 26-29
   — injection timing for travellers, 130
   — maximum effects of, 94
   dose, 25
   — adjustments, 73-75, 78-79
      during keto-acidosis, 84
      in children, 153-4
   — after childbirth, 113
   — during pregnancy, 111
   — reduction before exercise, 93
   — time changes and, 129-31

how it is used, 26-29
in blood, how it works, 14-16
— rise and fall after food, 4, 14, 15
infusion pumps, 31, 223-4
injections, 22
— aids for the blind 106, 186
— drawing up, 170-80
— damage from, 185
— equipment, 169-70
— fear of, 184
— for small children, 144-6
— increasing number of, 79
— sites, 181
altering, 79
cleansing skin at, 185
in children, 145-6
infection at, 185
swelling and pain at, 185
— sloppiness over, 163
— source, 13
— technique, 170-83
— timing, 29
altering, 76-77
injector guns, 146, 184
reactions see Insulin
shelf-life, 127-8
spilling, 185
travel precautions over, 127
types, 23-25
— adjustments, 75-76
weight loss and, 56
Insulin-dependent diabetes
   causes, 6
   definition, 5
   guidelines for teachers, 225-6
   long-term complications, 95-106
   people at risk, 6
   pregnancy and, 110-15

symptoms, 9
Insurance, 120-1
  driving, 135
  for children, 161-2
Intelligence, effect of hypoglycaemia
  on, 150-1
Intrauterine device, 115
Islets of Langerhans, 13

J

Jobs
  acceptable, 117-18
  applying for, 118
  effect of diabetes on, 118-19
  first-time, 119
Juvenile diabetes see Insulin-dependent
  diabetes

K

Keto-acidosis
  avoiding, 81-82
  cause, 18
  fluid intake during, 82-83
  insulin dose adjustment during, 84
  symptoms, 18, 82
  tests during, 82
Keto-Diastix, 196
Ketones
  formation, 5, 18
  testing for, 72, 196
Ketosis see Keto-acidosis
Ketostix, 196
Kidney damage, 100

L

Labour, diabetes control during, 112
Life assurance, 120

M

Marriage, diabetes and, 107
Maturity-onset diabetes see Non-insulin-
  dependent diabetes
Meals
  see also Diet; Food; Snacks
  effect of irregular, 86-87
  for children while travelling, 161
  late breakfast, 77
  late evening, 76-77, 132
  school, 154, 155
  size of, 38, 151
  timing, 30-31, 37-38
Meat, 220
  products, 50
Medical assistance abroad, 129
Medicines see Drugs
Menstruation, 109
Metabolism, normal, 12
Milk, 48
  exchange values, 41, 219
  products, 48, 219
Minerals in food, 36
Motor insurance, 120
Mountaineering, 124

N

Nail cutting, 97
Needles
  blocked, 187
  disposable, 187
  disposal of, 188
Neuritis, 95
  painful, 100
Neuropathy, 95
Non-insulin-dependent diabetes
  causes, 7

definition, 5
people at risk, 7
symptoms, 9
Nuts, 221

O

Operations, 104

P

Pain at injection site, 185
Pancreas, 13
   disease causing diabetes, 7
Parties, 132-3
   for children, 151-2
Pasta, 44
Pensions, 121
Pill, the contraceptive, 115-16
   causing diabetes, 8
Portions see Exchanges
Pregnancy, 108-9
   diabetes control after, 113
   diabetes control during, 111-12
   diabetes developing during, 111
Prescription charges, 121
Processed foods, 41, 218
Protein, foods containing, 35-36, 45, 46
Puberty, 108

R

Reactions, insulin see hypoglycaemia
Renal threshold of blood sugar, 16
Research into diabetes, 141
Retinal damage, 99
Rice, wholegrain, 44
Rock climbing, 124

S

School
   coping at, 154-9
   guidelines for teachers, 225-6
Seasonings, 46
Sexual development, 108
Sexual intercourse, 108
Shoes, 97-98
Sickness insurance, 121
   see also Illness
Skin cleaning at injection site, 185
Slimming see Weight loss
Smoking effects, 101, 137
Snacks
   effect of missed, 87
   importance of, 37
   timing, 31
Social life, 132-3
   eating out, 55-56
   teenagers, 164-5
Social Security help, 121
Sports see Exercise
Starch see carbohydrate
   in foods, 34, 209
   storage, 11
Statistics of diabetes, 1
Sterilization, 116
Stress
   effects in children, 158
   effects on blood sugar, 62,79
Sugar
   blood see Blood sugar
   foods containing, 34-35, 51-52
   in urine, 16-17
   — testing for see Urine tests
   substitutes, 46, 53, 54

Superannuation, 121
Sweeteners, 46, 53, 54
Swelling at injection site, 146, 185
Swimming, 123, 124
Symptoms
    in diabetes, 9, 17
    in hypoglycaemia, 80
    in keto-acidosis, 18, 82
Syringes
    disposable, 187
    disposal of, 188
    drawing up insulin into, 170-80
    for blind people, 106
    glass, 187
    travel precautions for, 127

T

Teacher guidelines for diabetes, 225-6
Teeth see Dentistry
Tests for sugar (general; also Blood tests;
    Urine tests)
    adjustments following, 74-80
    blood vs urine, 64
    effects of failing to perform, 163-4
    high evening, 75
    high mid-day and low evening, 76
    high morning, 74
    in children, 152-3
    low mid-day, 78
    menstruation and, 109
    need for, 63
    travel and, 131
Thirst, 17
Tiredness, 17
Toenail cutting, 97
Travel
    children and, 161-2

coping with, 125-32
help with cost of, 121
informing your friends, 126
insurance, 121
overseas
sickness, 126, 161
Triglyceride storage, 11

U

Urine
    excess passing of, 17
    sugar in, 16-17
Urine tests, 189-96
    see also Tests for sugar
    aids for blind people, 106
    at school, 158
    during keto-acidosis, 82, 84
    equipment, 189
    frequency, 71
    interpretation, 69
    misleading, 71-72
    timing, 71
    types, 70-71
    — Clinistix, 189
    — Clinitest, 70, 189
    — Diabur — Test 5000, 70, 195
    — Diastix, 70, 193
    — Keto-Diastix, 196
    — Ketostix, 196

V

Vaccinations, 126
    for children, 162
Vasectomy, 116
Vegetables, 43, 44, 46
    exchange values, 41, 213, 216
Visidex II test, 65, 199

Vision
    blurring from high blood sugar, 20
    deterioration, 98-99

W

Weakness, 17
Weight gain in children, 157
Weight loss, 17
    insulin and, 56
Weights and measures, 222

Y

Yoghurt, 48, 219

The British Diabetic Association (BDA) was formed in 1934 to help all diabetics, to overcome prejudice and ignorance about diabetes, and to raise money for research.

The Association provides practical guidance and information on all aspects of living with diabetes (see page 139).

For over 50 years, the BDA has strived to achieve its aims, but has only been able to move forward with the continued support of its members and supporters. The BDA's authority comes from the size of its membership — the more members, the greater its influence on their behalf.

To become a member, fill in the application form and send it with your subscription to:

The British Diabetic Association
10 Queen Anne Street
London W1M 0BD

Enrolment Form

British Diabetic Association
10 Queen Anne Street
London W1M 0BD

MEMBERSHIP SUBSCRIPTIONS

Life membership	Single payment of £105 or £15 a year for 7 years under covenant
Annual membership	£5.00 a year
Pensioner, student on government grant and those in receipt of DSS benefits.	£1.00 a year
Overseas annual membership	£10.00 a year
Overseas life membership	Single payment of £150.00

Please enrol me as a:

☐ Life member: £105 £15 a year for 7 years under covenant

☐ Annual member: £5.00

☐ Reduced rate membership: £1.00

☐ Overseas annual member: £10.00

☐ Overseas Life member: £150.00

☐ Are you joining on behalf of a child? (Children in the UK under the age of 16 can join free for one year if they wish)

I enclose Remittance/Banker's Order/Covenant for £..........................
(Please delete whichever does not apply)

Date.. Signature ....

Full name: Mr/Mrs/Miss..
(Block Capitals please)

Address ....

....

Date of Birth.............................. Occupation ....
(This information will be treated as strictly confidential)